Health Systems in Transition

Mexico

Health System Review 2020

Miguel Á González Block

Hortensia Reyes Morales

Lucero Cahuana Hurtado

Alejandra Balandrán

Edna Méndez

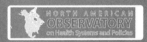
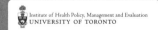
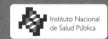

The North American Observatory on Health Systems and Policies (NAO) is a collaborative partnership of interested researchers, academic organizations, governments, and health organizations. Through its work, the NAO promotes evidence-informed health system policy decision-making in Canada, Mexico, and the United States of America at the national and the subnational levels of government. Academic partners include the Institute of Health Policy Management and Evaluation at the Dalla Lana School of Public Health, University of Toronto, the National Institute of Public Health, Mexico, and the UCLA Fielding School of Public Health.

The European Observatory on Health Systems and Policies supports and promotes evidence-based health policy-making through comprehensive and rigorous analysis of health systems in Europe. It brings together a wide range of policy-makers, academics and practitioners to analyse trends in health reform, drawing on experience from across Europe to illuminate policy issues. This Health System in Transition profile is the result of collaboration between the NAO and the European Observatory on Health Systems and Policies. The Observatory is a partnership, hosted by WHO/Europe, with a secretariat in Brussels and hubs in London (at the London School of Economics and Political Science and the London School of Hygiene & Tropical Medicine) and at the Berlin University of Technology.

UNIVERSITY OF TORONTO PRESS

Toronto Buffalo London

Published by the WHO Regional Office for Europe acting as host organization for, and secretariat of, the European Observatory on Health Systems and Policies under the title *Health Systems in Transition: Mexico*. 2020.

© World Health Organization 2020, on behalf of the European Observatory on Health Systems and Policies

The Regional Office for Europe of the World Health Organization has granted reproduction and electronic publishing rights to University of Toronto Press.

Published in North America by University of Toronto Press, 2021
Toronto Buffalo London
utorontopress.com
Printed in the U.S.A.

ISBN 978-1-4875-0852-4 (paper)   ISBN 978-1-4875-3843-9 (EPUB)   ISBN 978-1-4875-3842-2 (PDF)

Publication cataloguing information is available from Library and Archives Canada.

Please address requests about the publication to
Publications,
WHO Regional Office for Europe
UN City,
Marmorvej 51,
DK-2100 Copenhagen Ø, Denmark

Alternatively, complete an online request form for documentation, health information, or for permission to quote or translate, on the Regional Office website (http://www.euro.who.int/pubrequest).

The views expressed by authors or editors do not necessarily represent the decisions or the stated policies of the European Observatory on Health Systems and Policies or any of its partners.

The designations employed and the presentation of the material in this publication do not imply the expression of any opinion whatsoever on the part of the European Observatory on Health Systems and Policies or any of its partners concerning the legal status of any country, territory, city, or area of its authorities, or concerning the delimitation of its frontiers or boundaries. Where the designation "country or area" appears in the headings of tables, it covers countries, territories, cities, or areas. Dotted lines on maps represent approximate border lines for which there may not yet be full agreement.

The mention of specific companies or of certain manufacturers' products does not imply that they are endorsed or recommended by the European Observatory on Health Systems and Policies in preference to others of a similar nature that are not mentioned. Errors and omissions are excepted, the names of proprietary products are distinguished by initial capital letters.

The European Observatory on Health Systems and Policies does not warrant that the information contained in this publication is complete and correct and shall not be liable for any damages incurred as a result of its use.

University of Toronto Press acknowledges the financial assistance to its publishing program of the Canada Council for the Arts and the Ontario Arts Council, an agency of the Government of Ontario.

**Canada Council
for the Arts**   **Conseil des Arts
du Canada**

ONTARIO ARTS COUNCIL
CONSEIL DES ARTS DE L'ONTARIO
an Ontario government agency
un organisme du gouvernement de l'Ontario

Funded by the
Government
of Canada   Financé par le
gouvernement
du Canada

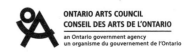

CONTENTS

Preface · vii

Acknowledgements · ix

List of abbreviations · xi

List of tables, figures and boxes · xv

Abstract · xix

Executive summary · xxi

1 Introduction · 1
 1.1 *Geography and sociodemography* · 1
 1.2 *Economic context* · 4
 1.3 *Political context* · 6
 1.4 *Health status* · 9

2 Organization and governance · 17
 2.1 *Historical background* · 18
 2.2 *Organization* · 32
 2.3 *Decentralization and centralization* · 43
 2.4 *Intersectorality* · 45
 2.5 *Health information systems* · 47
 2.6 *Regulation and planning* · 49
 2.7 *Person-centred care* · 68

3 Financing · 77
 3.1 *Health expenditure* · 78
 3.2 *Sources of revenue and financing flows* · 86
 3.3 *Overview of the statutory financing system* · 88
 3.4 *Out-of-pocket health expenses* · 92
 3.5 *Voluntary health insurance* · 94
 3.6 *Other sources of financing* · 97
 3.7 *Payment mechanisms* · 97

4   Physical and human resources — 99
4.1 *Physical resources* — 100
4.2 *Human resources* — 110

5   Provision of services — 124
5.1 *Public health* — 125
5.2 *Patient pathways* — 132
5.3 *Primary/ambulatory care* — 135
5.4 *Specialized outpatient care/hospital care* — 136
5.5 *Emergency care* — 141
5.6 *Pharmaceutical care* — 143
5.7 *Rehabilitation and intermediate care* — 148
5.8 *Long-term care* — 150
5.9 *Care by informal caregivers* — 151
5.10 *Palliative care* — 151
5.11 *Mental health* — 153
5.12 *Dental care* — 156
5.13 *Complementary and alternative medicine* — 156

6   Principal health reforms — 158
6.1 *The System for Social Protection in Health* — 159
6.2 *Financial impact of SPSS* — 160
6.3 *Equity and efficiency impacts of SPSS* — 163
6.4 *Demand-side funding by SPSS* — 165
6.5 *Portability and convergence* — 166
6.6 *Persistence of segmentation* — 168
6.7 *Future developments* — 169

7   Assessment of the health system — 175
7.1 *Health system governance* — 176
7.2 *Accessibility* — 179
7.3 *Financial protection* — 181
7.4 *Health care quality* — 184
7.5 *Health system outcomes* — 185
7.6 *Health system efficiency* — 187

8   Conclusions — 190

Postscript: Response to the COVID-19 pandemic — 195

9 Appendices   200

9.1 *References*   200

9.2 *Useful websites*   218

9.3 *HiT methodology and production process*   218

9.4 *The review process*   221

9.5 *About the authors*   221

Index   223

The Health Systems in Transition (HiT) series consists of country-based reviews that provide a detailed description of a health system and of reform and policy initiatives in progress or under development in a specific country. Each review is produced by country experts in collaboration with staff at the North American Observatory on Health Systems and Policies and the European Observatory on Health Systems and Policies. In order to facilitate comparisons between countries, reviews are based on a template prepared by the European Observatory, which is revised periodically. The template provides detailed guidelines and specific questions, definitions and examples needed to compile a report.

HiTs seek to provide relevant information to support policy-makers and analysts in the development of health systems. They are building blocks that can be used to:

- learn in detail about different approaches to the organization, financing and delivery of health services, and the role of the main actors in health systems;
- describe the institutional framework, process, content and imple-mentation of health care reform programmes;
- highlight challenges and areas that require more in-depth analysis;
- provide a tool for the dissemination of information on health systems and the exchange of experiences of reform strategies between policy-makers and analysts in different countries; and
- assist other researchers in more in-depth comparative health policy analysis.

Compiling the reviews poses a number of methodological problems. In many countries, there is relatively little information available on the health system and the impact of reforms. Due to the lack of a uniform data source, quantitative data on health services are based on a number of different sources, including data from national statistical offices, the Organisation for Economic Co-operation and Development (OECD), the International Monetary Fund (IMF), the World Bank's World Development Indicators and any other relevant sources considered useful by the authors. Data collection methods and definitions sometimes vary, but typically are consistent within each separate review.

A standardized review has certain disadvantages because the financing and delivery of health care differ across countries. However, it also offers advantages because it raises similar issues and questions. HiTs can be used to inform policy-makers about experiences in other countries that may be relevant to their own national situations. They can also be used to inform comparative analysis of health systems. This series is an ongoing initiative and material is updated at regular intervals.

Comments and suggestions for the further development and improvement of the HiT series are most welcome and can be sent to info@obs.euro.who.int.

HiTs and HiT summaries are available on the Observatory's website (http://www.healthobservatory.eu).

ACKNOWLEDGEMENTS

The Health Systems in Transition (HiT) profile on Mexico was co-produced by the North American Observatory on Health Systems and Policies (NAO) and the European Observatory on Health Systems and Policies.

The North American Observatory on Health Systems and Policies is a collaborative partnership of interested researchers, governments and health organizations promoting evidence-informed health system decision-making with academic directors in Canada, Mexico and the United States of America. The NAO partnership secretariat is hosted by the Institute of Health Policy, Management & Evaluation at the University of Toronto.

The European Observatory is a partnership that includes the Governments of Austria, Belgium, Finland, Ireland, Norway, Slovenia, Sweden, Switzerland and the United Kingdom; the Veneto Region of Italy; the French National Union of Health Insurance Funds (UNCAM); the World Health Organization; the European Commission; the World Bank; the London School of Economics and Political Science (LSE); and the London School of Hygiene & Tropical Medicine (LSHTM). The partnership is hosted by the WHO Regional Office for Europe.

This edition was written by Miguel Á González Block, Hortensia Reyes Morales, Lucero Cahuana Hurtado, Alejandra Balandrán and Edna Méndez. It was edited by Sara Allin and Gregory Marchildon, University of Toronto and NAO, who also contributed to the text. Thanks are given to Beatriz Martínez Zavala for her editorial and research support.

The NAO is grateful to Arturo Bustamante, University of California, Los Angeles, and Eduardo Álvarez Falcón, Proxture, for reviewing the manuscript. The authors are also grateful to Dr Adolfo Martínez Valle, Universidad Nacional Autónoma de México, formerly at Dirección General de Evaluación del Desempeño, Secretaría de Salud, Mexico, for his assistance in providing information and for his comments on previous drafts of the manuscript and suggestions about plans and current policy options in the Mexican health system. The authors thank the NAO for providing the research funds necessary to organize and prepare the first draft of this HiT. The authors also appreciated the substantive editing by Sara Allin and Gregory Marchildon and the copy-editing work of Patrick Farrell, and the editorial staff at the European Observatory.

Thanks are also extended to World Bank and OECD for the data on health financing and services. This HiT reflects the organization of the health system and the data availability, unless otherwise indicated, as it was in December, 2019.

The North American Observatory HiT series is coordinated by Gregory Marchildon and Sara Allin. The production and copy-editing process was coordinated within the European Observatory by Jonathan North with the support of Elizabeth Hoile.

AMFEM	Mexican Association of Faculties and Schools of Medicine
AMH	Mexican Association of Hospitals
AMI	Acute myocardial infarction
AMIIF	Mexican Association of Innovative Pharmaceutical Industry
ANM	National Academy of Medicine
ANUIES	National Association of Universities and Institutions of Higher Education
ASE	State government solidary contribution
ASF	Federal solidary contribution
CAF	Consultation rooms adjacent to pharmacy offices
CAUSES	Universal Health Services Catalogue
CBDH	National Commission for Human Rights
CCPNMIS	Coordinating Commission for Negotiating the Price of Medicines and other Health Inputs
CENETEC	National Centre of Technological Excellence in Health
CENSIDA	National Centre for the Prevention and Control of HIV/AIDS
CETIFARMA	Council for Ethics and Transparency of the Pharmaceutical Industry
CFM	Mexican Pharmaceutical Consortium
CIFRHS	Interinstitutional Commission for the Training of Human Resources for Health
CINSHAE	National Commission for National Institutes of Health and High Specialty Hospitals
CLUES	Unique Health Establishment Code
CNPSS	Commission for Social Protection in Health
CNSF	National Insurance and Securities Commission
COFECE	Federal Commission for Economic Competition
COFEPRIS	Federal Commission for the Protection Against Sanitary Risks
CONACEM	Committee for Medical Specialty Councils
CONACYT	National Science and Technology Council

CONALEP	National Council of Technical Professional Education
CONAMED	National Commission for Medical Arbitration
CONAPO	National Council on Population
CONASUPO	National Company for Subsidies for the Population
CONEVAL	National Council for the Evaluation of Social Development Policy
COPLAMAR	General Coordination of the National Plan for Depressed Zones and Marginalized Groups
CPG	Clinical practice guideline
CT	Computed tomography
DGCES	General Directorate for Health Quality and Education
DGED	General Directorate for Performance Evaluation
DGIS	General Directorate for Health Information
DGPLADES	General Directorate for Health Planning and Development
DIF	National System for Integral Family Development
DMTDI	Directorate for Traditional Medicine and Intercultural Development
DRG	Diagnostic Related Groups
EAP	Economically active population
ECE	Electronic health records
EMR	Electronic medical record
ENARM	National Exam for Medical Residency Candidates
ENOE	National Occupation and Employment Surveys
ENSANUT	National Health and Nutrition Survey
FASSA	Health Services Contribution Fund
FCS	Carlos Slim Foundation
FFS	Fee-for-service
FPGC	Protection Fund for Catastrophic Health Expenditures
Funsalud	Mexican Health Foundation
GBD	Global Burden of Disease Study
GDP	Gross Domestic Product
GHC	General Health Council
GHL	General Health Law
HAI	Health Care Associated Infections
HDI	Human Development Index
IMR	Infant mortality rate
IMSS	Mexican Social Insurance Institute

INAPAM	National Institute for Older Persons
INEGI	National Institute of Statistics and Geography
INSABI	Institute for Health for Wellbeing
INSS	National Institute of Social Insurance
ISES	Special Health Insurance Institutions
ISS	Social Services Institute
ISSSTE	Institute for Social Security and Services for State Employees
MoH	Ministry of Health
Morena	Movement for National Regeneration Party
MRI	Magnetic resonance imaging
NAFTA	North American Free Trade Agreement
NGO	Nongovernmental organization
NHS	National Health System
OECD	Organisation for Economic Co-operation and Development
OIC	Organs for Internal Control
PABI	Self-Regulation of Food and Non-Alcoholic Drink Advertisement Directed to Child Audiences
PAE	Specific Action Programmes
PAHO	Pan American Health Organization
PAN	National Action Party
PEF	Federal Expenditure Budget
PEMEX	Mexican Petroleum Company
PET	Positron emission tomography
PMI	Master Plan for Physical Infrastructure for Health
PPP	Purchase power parity
PRI	Institutional Revolutionary Party
REPSS	State Regimens for Social Protection in Health
RHOVE	Hospital Epidemiological Surveillance Network
SEMAR	Secretariat of the Navy
SiNaCEAM	National System for Certification of Medical Care Establishments
SINAIS	National Health Information System
SINAVE	National Epidemiological Surveillance System
SINBA	National Basic Health Information System
SNPSS	Sistema Nacional de Protección Social en Salud. National System for Social Protection in Health

SPSS	System for Social Protection in Health
SRCV	Retirement, Cessation in Old Age and Old Age Insurance
SSA	Ministry of Health and Assistance
SUIVE	Unique Epidemiological Surveillance Information System
UMA	Unit for Measurement and Updating
UMF	Family Medicine Unit
UNEME	Specialized Medical Unit
USMBHA	US–Mexico Border Health Association
VSRS	Leave Healthy, Return Healthy Program
WHO	World Health Organization
YLPD	Years of life lost due to premature death

LIST OF TABLES, FIGURES AND BOXES

■ Tables

TABLE 1.1 Population and demographic indicators, 1991–2017   3

TABLE 1.2 Macroeconomic indicators for Mexico, 2000–2017   6

TABLE 1.3 Mortality and health indicators for Mexico, 1990–2017   10

TABLE 1.4 Mortality rates in Mexico by selected causes, 1990–2015   12

TABLE 1.5 Risk factors related to health in Mexico, 2005 or earliest year and 2017 or latest year   15

TABLE 1.6 Selected disease morbidity rates in Mexico, 2005 and 2017   16

TABLE 2.1 IMSS insurance according to regimen, contribution modality and benefit scheme, 2014   40

TABLE 2.2 Responsibilities for specific health system functions according to levels of care in the Mexican health system   50

TABLE 2.3 Situation of patient rights in Mexico   71

TABLE 3.1 Trends in health expenditure in Mexico, 2000–2015   81

TABLE 3.2 Percentage distribution of total expenditure on health by health function and financing scheme, 2015   85

TABLE 3.3 Public health expenditure on health by service input, 2010 and 2015 (%)   85

TABLE 3.4 Provider payment mechanisms   97

TABLE 4.1 Hospital units in the Mexican health system by institution, 2003 and 2015/2018   103

TABLE 4.2 Hospital beds in the Mexican health system by institution and year, 2003 and 2015/2018   104

TABLE 4.3 Public sector hospital beds per 100 000 inhabitants at state level, 2000, 2010 and 2014   105

TABLE 4.4 Hospital beds in acute hospitals per 1000 population in Mexico, OECD countries and Brazil, 2000, 2010 and 2016a   107

TABLE 4.5 CT and MRI equipment per million inhabitants in Mexico, compared with other countries in Latin America and OECD average, 2016   108

TABLE 4.6 Health workforce for selected categories according to information source, sector of employment and density, 2016   113

TABLE 4.7 Graduates in health sciences, 2011 and 2017   120

TABLE 5.1 Principal strengths and weaknesses of primary care services in Mexico   137

TABLE 5.2 National firms of allopathic, homeopathic or herbal medicines with a health licence   144

TABLE 5.3 Main organizations grouping drug dispensers in Mexico   145

TABLE 5.4 Palliative care services in Mexico, 2012   152

TABLE 6.1 Five financial imbalances motivating the SPSS, 2000 and 2014   161

■ Figures

FIG. 1.1 Political division of the country (32 states)   3

FIG. 2.1 Organization of the Mexican health system according to funding, provision and population coverage   33

FIG. 3.1 Total health expenditures as a share (%) of GDP in OECD countries, 2018   78

FIG. 3.2 Trends in health spending as a share (%) of GDP in Mexico and selected countries, 2000–2015   79

FIG. 3.3 Total health expenditures in US$ PPP per capita in OECD countries, 2018   80

FIG. 3.4 Public expenditure on health as a share (%) of current health expenditure in OECD countries, 2018   83

FIG. 3.5 Public expenditure on health as a share (%) of government expenditure in OECD countries, 2018 or latest available data   84

FIG. 3.6 Financial flows for the payment of health providers, 2020   88

FIG. 3.7 Coverage of the public health system in Mexico, 2018   89

FIG. 3.8 Magnitude and composition of annual household out-of-pocket expenses by socioeconomic level, 2016   94

FIG. 4.1 General physicians per 10 000 inhabitants by state, 2005 and 2014   114

FIG. 4.2 General physicians in Mexico, 2005–2014   115

FIG. 4.3 Distribution of medical specialists per 10 000 inhabitants, by state, 2005 and 2014   117

FIG. 4.4 Specialized physicians, 2005–2014   117

FIG. 4.5 Practising nurses and physicians per 1000 population, 2016 or latest   118

FIG. 5.1 Perceived quality indicators, National Health System, 2003–2017   140

FIG. 7.1 Proportion (%) of households reporting catastrophic and impoverishing health expenditures, 1992–2012   181

FIG. 7.2 Healthcare Access and Quality (HAQ) Index, Mexico and selected countries, 2016   183

FIG. 7.3 Healthcare Access and Quality (HAQ) Index, Mexico, by state, 2016   183

FIG. 7.4 Expenditure on health and life expectancy at birth (years), Mexico and selected OECD countries, 2000–2015   187

■ Boxes

BOX 5.1 Model patterns of access to medical care   133

BOX 5.2 Efforts to improve integration of care   139

BOX 6.1 High-specialty exchange agreements   167

ABSTRACT

This analysis of the Mexican health system reviews recent developments in organization and governance, health financing, health care provision, health reforms and health system performance. The Mexican health system consists of three main components operating in parallel: 1) employment-based social insurance schemes, 2) public assistance services for the uninsured supported by a financial protection scheme, and 3) a private sector composed of service providers, insurers, and pharmaceutical and medical device manufacturers and distributors. The social insurance schemes are managed by highly centralized national institutions while coverage for the uninsured is operated by both state and federal authorities and providers. The largest social insurance institution – the Mexican Social Insurance Institute (IMSS) – is governed by a corporatist arrangement, which reflects the political realities of the 1940s rather than the needs of the 21st century. National health spending has grown in recent years but is lower than the Latin America and Caribbean average and considerably lower than the OECD average in 2015. Public spending accounts for 58% of total financing, with private contributions being mostly comprised of out-of-pocket spending. The private sector, while regulated by the government, mostly operates independently. Mexico's health system delivers a wide range of health care services; however, nearly 14% of the population lacks financial protection, while the insured are mostly enrolled in diverse public schemes which provide varying benefits packages. Private sector services are in high demand given insufficient resources among most public institutions and the lack of voice by the insured to ensure the fulfilment of entitlements. Furthermore, the system faces challenges with obesity, diabetes, violence, as well as with health inequity. Recognizing the inequities in access created by its segmented structure, both civil society and government are calling for greater integration of service delivery across public institutions, although no consensus yet exists as to how to bring this about.

EXECUTIVE SUMMARY

■ Mexico faces challenges with income inequality, health inequities and a range of health concerns such as obesity, diabetes, mental illness and some infectious diseases

Mexico is a federation consisting of 32 states including Mexico City. It is the 15th largest country geographically and 11th most populous country in the world with over 124 million residents, of whom 77% live in urban areas. The population is young, with nearly 27% under the age of 15, and only 7% who are 65 years and older. The fertility rate has declined steadily since the 1990s, and educational attainment is gradually increasing (88% completing high school in 2015 up from 77%). Indigenous Peoples and people who recognize themselves as afrodescendants make up about 12% and 1% of the population, respectively, and face a disproportionate burden of health and social challenges.

Income inequality and poverty are persistent health challenges. Of the 36 countries making up the OECD, Mexico has the highest level of income inequality. Poverty disproportionately affects rural residents: in 2016 about 58% of Mexico's rural residents were facing poverty, compared with 39% of the urban population.

Life expectancy in Mexico increased rapidly over the course of the last century, but, at nearly 75 years in 2017, it remains lower than most other OECD countries. While mortality rates have declined over the past 20 years, there is a big gap between men and women, and the infant mortality rate is above that of Argentina, Chile, Costa Rica and Cuba. The main causes of death in 2015 in the general population were diabetes and ischaemic heart disease, both conditions having increased significantly since 1990, followed by homicide (among men), which has been relatively stable over this time.

Obesity – one of the main risk factors for diabetes and heart disease – is a very significant health concern. Mexico ranks second highest in the world in overall prevalence of obesity (behind only the United States), and highest in the world for overweight and obese children. Additional challenges relate to food insecurity, which affects about 28% of households, as well as acute malnutrition and anaemia in children, lower respiratory infections and acute diarrhoeal disease. Smoking and alcohol consumption are relatively low compared with other OECD countries, yet related conditions such as chronic obstructive pulmonary diseases and alcohol cirrhosis are among the top 10 causes of premature death and disability.

Mexico's health system is segmented across diverse public and private payers and providers

Social insurance is provided by highly centralized, national institutions, while voluntary coverage for the uninsured was, until 2020, operated by both state and federal authorities and providers. The private sector, while regulated by government, operates mostly independently.

Mexico's health system is thus segmented across diverse public and private payers and providers and is organized under national or federal public institutions and by private providers and insurers. Since 1982, the federal Ministry of Health (MoH) coordinates the National Health System (NHS), a notion enacted in the General Health Law that relates all public and private payers and providers to the MoH through varying modalities and degrees of authority.

The social insurance subsystem is dominated by three national institutions that cover all salaried employees in the formal sector. The IMSS covers private sector employees and the Institute for Social Security and Services for State Employees (ISSSTE) covers federal government employees. In 2017, IMSS covered about 33% and ISSSTE 7.4% of the population, respectively. Both IMSS and ISSSTE organize, provide and regulate most of their own health services through vertically integrated, national organizations. However, a significant proportion of affiliates seek care outside social insurance institutions to get around access barriers or to access higher quality services. State governments fund health services for their civil servants primarily through their own social insurance institutes or through agreements with either

ISSSTE or IMSS. In addition to IMSS, ISSSTE and MoH institutions, there are individual insurance funds for dedicated populations such as the military, navy and the oil company Petróleos Mexicanos (PEMEX), which all respectively fund and provide health services for their forces and employees.

The MoH and state governments and their health provider networks share responsibility for public health programmes for the entire population, health coverage and social assistance for the uninsured poor, and financial protection for the self-employed and for those employed in the informal labour market. The MoH is the main health care funder for health services for the uninsured and is also the main provider of specialty hospital services, while state health provider networks provide primary and general hospital care. Seguro Popular – the major financial protection scheme for those outside social insurance arrangements and the unemployed – covered up until the phasing out of SPSS 43.5% of the population, providing them with a broad yet limited package of health benefits. Health services are provided mostly by MoH at state and federal levels, often with access and quality limitations in spite of funding efforts by Seguro Popular and now by the Institute for Health for Wellbeing (INSABI) that replaced it. Those not covered by Seguro Popular (now INSABI) and even those protected by other health insurance programmes are able to pay out-of-pocket to use MoH hospitals and state medical facilities according to a scale related to income.

Funding for health services for Mexicans not protected by a social insurance programme is mostly through the MoH and state governments, and was channelled directly to federal hospitals and state providers through SPSS, which outlined a set of laws and rules to establish a mix of historical-based funding, capitation and activity-based funding. Federal hospitals are funded through historical budgets and case-based reimbursement. State providers for the uninsured are funded by the federal and state governments based on the number of people registered with with SPSS and now INSABI. Under SPSS, about half of this funding was transferred on the basis of historical budgets, with the other half paid based on performance agreements or activity-based funding. SPSS was operated through the National Commission for Social Protection in Health (CNPSS), a decentralized, arm's-length MoH organ, supported at the state level by a decentralized State Regimens for Social Protection in Health (REPSS). REPSS were at arm's length from state health providers and state authorities, thus enabling more transparent and accountable use of federal and state funds.

Private health insurance covers nearly 8% of the population, many of whom are higher-income individuals who are also covered by IMSS or ISSSTE and receive private insurance as a benefit through their employer. Private practice is highly fragmented and most private services are paid out-of-pocket on a fee-for-services basis.

In 2018, 13.6% of the population – approximately 17.8 million people – did not have any public financial protection coverage to enable them to make use of public health services free of charge, and likely did not have private insurance either. About half of the uninsured are middle class self-employed people who choose not to enrol in Seguro Popular.

The populations protected by social insurance and Seguro Popular and now by INSABI are, however, highly mobile. Between January and December of 2014, up to 38% of those insured by IMSS ceased employment for periods longer than 2 months and as a result lost their coverage by IMSS medical facilities. Of this group, 61.2% found employment outside the formal private sector, of whom 11.3% became government employees and therefore became protected by ISSSTE or a state employee health insurer. The rest could have registered with Seguro Popular or chosen to maintain their IMSS coverage as dependents of an insured person.

The federal government regulates health providers and funders as well as firms involved in the manufacture, distribution and sale of medical inputs and pharmaceuticals and in private health insurance. Regulation is divided across the MoH, the National Insurance and Securities Commission (CNSF) and the General Health Council (GHC) – an entity that reports directly to the president. The GHC is in charge of voluntary facility accreditation as well as registering medical devices and pharmaceuticals prior to being considered for inclusion in each public institution's basic input lists. Such lists consist of institutionally approved pharmaceuticals and medical devices that are both approved by the GHC and considered necessary and affordable by each institution. The GHC is also empowered to declare national health emergencies, this being the chief reason for its subordination to the presidency. Social insurance health providers are self-regulated.

Health professionals are trained in 155 medical schools and faculties although only 103 are overseen and accredited by the Mexican Association of Faculties and Schools of Medicine (AMFEM), a private, voluntary organization. The Ministry of Education licenses and registers medical faculties and schools, as well as graduates, but has no authority to set limits to the number of medical students enrolled. State and national medical colleges and specialty councils regulate professional practice, which is obligatory for specialists, who must be reaccredited every 5 years, but not for general physicians.

■ Public spending on health has grown in recent years but out-of-pocket payments remain a significant source of health care expenditure

Total health expenditure in Mexico as a share of GDP was 5.7% in 2015, which is lower than the Latin American and the Caribbean average and considerably lower than the OECD average. Health spending growth has been significant since 2000, when Mexico spent US$ 480.50 (adjusting for differences in purchasing power (PPP) per capita), a figure that more than doubled in 2015, becoming US$ 1 009 (PPP) in real terms.

Public spending on health as a percentage of total health expenditure increased between 2000 and 2015, from 43.7% to 53.8%. This is partly a response to the implementation of the SPSS, which contributed to reducing out-of-pocket spending from 53.9% of total health expenditure in 2000 to 41.3% in 2015. However, out-of-pocket spending continues to be a major source of financing in the country, placing Mexico well above the OECD average (19% of total health expenditure). Just under half of public health spending is directed towards outpatient care, and a third funds hospital services.

The segmentation of the country's health system corresponds to these diverse sources of financing. Social insurance is financed through employee and employer contributions and government subsidies. In 2015, 30% of total health expenditure was from social insurance, although it covers over 42% of the population. Public health services are financed by taxes and government revenues. The SPSS, which financed Seguro Popular, made up 24% of total health expenditure in 2015. Its financing emulates that of other social insurance institutions, as it is made up of federal, state and family contributions. Voluntary private health insurance plays only a minor role and accounts for under 5% of spending.

Despite the fact that public health care providers offer a broad range of services – particularly so among social insurance institutions – problems such as long wait times, lack of trust and the unavailability of medicines forces many to use private providers, resulting in out-of-pocket expenses. The probability of a person incurring out-of-pocket expenses is high even when public health insurance is available.

■ Human resources and physical infrastructure are in relatively low supply compared with other OECD countries, and are unequally distributed across the country

Mexico has a total of 230 922 physicians, at a rate of 1.9 per 1000 inhabitants; low compared with the OECD average of 3.3 per 1000 inhabitants. While up to 71% of general physicians are publicly employed, their density relative to the general population varies across states, from 0.6 per 1000 inhabitants in the State of Mexico to 1.8 per 1000 inhabitants in Mexico City. Mexico has just above 342 000 nurses, with professional nurses numbering just below 198 000, and the remainder being technical personnel with high school educations. Nurse density is 2.8 per 1000 inhabitants, one third lower than the OECD average.

Among over 21 000 primary care units operated by public institutions, 67.3% belong to the MoH and 20% to the IMSS-Bienestar programme, while IMSS owns 5.2% and ISSSTE, 4.8%. A total of 6735 private primary care facilities are registered, of which 5844 are consulting rooms adjacent to pharmacies. However, close to 60 000 private medical offices have been registered by economic statistics as generally offering the services of a single professional, mostly general or specialized physicians.

Mexico has a total of 4341 hospitals, of which 1381 (30%) are public and are generally larger than the private hospitals, which total 2960. Hospitals catering for the insured account for 39% of the total in the public sector while those for the non-insured – generally smaller – account for 61% of the total. Hospitals are concentrated in urban areas, with only 46 (3.3%) located in rural localities. The majority of Mexico's 2960 private sector hospitals are smaller establishments, with only 94 providing 50 beds or more. Total bed density across hospitals is 1.56 per 1000 inhabitants, or 0.76 considering only public beds. Among public hospitals in Mexico City, density is 1.8 beds per 1000 inhabitants. Bed density decreased by 4.5% at the national level between 2000 and 2014.

Hospital care is offered by each institution and private provider according to their own infrastructure and levels of care, generally distinguishing between general (second level) and highly specialized (third level) hospitals. Private hospitals represent 24.3% of beds and are responsible for 25.1% of hospital discharges in the country.

Mexico has a shortage of high-cost medical technology. For example, magnetic resonance imaging (MRI) machines per million inhabitants is 2.6 compared with 6.8 in Brazil and 15.6 OECD average. Similar levels exist with respect to gamma cameras and radiation therapy equipment, while access to mammograph equipment is just 42.5% compared with the OECD average.

■ Mexico's health system delivers a broad range of care services but not all are publicly funded and available without out-of-pocket payments

The MoH funds, coordinates and conducts countrywide disease prevention activities through health promotion, education and epidemiological surveillance. Health authorities at the state level are responsible for the local coordination and implementation of public health activities. Social insurance institutions also run disease prevention programmes, targeting similar priorities to those of the MoH, including chronic diseases, accident prevention, vaccination and neonatal screening.

Launched in 2015 and still in the early stages of implementation, the MoH's Comprehensive Health Care Model (MAIS) strategy aims to define and monitor patients' pathways through the health care system to ensure timely delivery of quality services. Primary care is delivered through the broad but still-limited network of the MoH, social insurance and private health care services, each of which operates within separate hierarchical networks. Public sector primary care facilities contribute to the provision of a wide range of services, including dental care, vaccination, family planning, prenatal care and paediatric care, as well as health promotion activities. In the private sector the focus of care is limited to curative medical care.

Neither the federal or state governments fund or otherwise provide day care services, although some day care support services are available in the private sector. However, the concept of day care is used when referring to social services supporting the elderly.

Emergency care is provided through the emergency services facilities at both public and private hospitals, which will accommodate patients regardless of their institutional coverage. Emergency services operate 24 hours a day, attended by general practitioners and specialists in medical emergencies in coordination with a broad network of first responders.

Mexico does not have an integrated pharmaceutical policy, but sectoral health programmes include strategies and action plans to improve access to medicines. The Mexican pharmaceutical industry ranks second in Latin America behind Brazil, and includes a total of 742 pharmaceutical companies in operation. The public sector procures medicines through approved lists and consolidated purchasing.

Care for the rehabilitation of patients with disabilities is mainly provided by public and private non-profit institutions. Intermediate care is provided by the MoH through a network of specialized units that aim at reducing hospitalizations. Long-term care is practically non-existent, while palliative care policies have only recently been developed. While informal caregivers are plentiful, they lack support and coordination within the health system. Mental health policy and services are undeveloped, with care concentrated in psychiatric hospitals in spite of efforts to develop community programmes.

■ The government faces challenges to attain universal coverage through increasing financing and expanding services for the uninsured while retaining the segmented health system

From 2000 up to at least 2018, health policy in Mexico was characterized by the pursuit of universal health coverage, as promised by the 1983 constitutional reform, while maintaining the segmented health system. President López Obrador's administration has promised to integrate the health system and end segmentation during its tenure from 2018 to 2024. However, no consensus yet exists as to how to bring this about.

Since 1983, reforms to national health policy have aimed to better integrate the segmented health system into a more coherent whole with the goal of attaining greater equity and efficiency for all Mexicans. A constitutional reform that year introduced a universal right to health protection but was limited in its capacity to empower the MoH with the ability to influence policy across existing social assistance and insurance institutions or the private sector. In 2011 the Constitution recognized the Right to Health as declared by the International Covenant on Economic, Social and Cultural Rights. However, the constitutional right to health protection as implemented by the General Health Law is limited to a set of coordination measures across federal institutions and with states. Among the most important reforms towards the implementation of the constitutional right to health was the 2003 establishment of SPSS, which involved both the federal and state governments, and the 2006 implementation of the Strategy for Portability and Convergence to promote the coordination and delivery of high specialty hospital services across social insurance and the MoH, regardless of institutional affiliation. More recently, in 2014, a reform was implemented to increase SPSS accountability.

The Mexican health system faces shortages and inconsistencies in health resources, problems that are growing in rural areas. Human resources shortages principally affect nurses and medical specialists as well as efforts to address health promotion and prevention through an intersectoral focus. The problem of a lack of medical specialists grows due to bottlenecks in training, early retirement in the public sector and the growth of chronic diseases that increasingly demand specialist skills. Resource imbalances particularly affect rural areas and small cities, where insecurity and lack of infrastructure are constant problems.

Beyond the need for more specialists, shortages also make it difficult for hospitals to provide access to technology and innovative medicines, which together with the rapid growth of chronic diseases makes the problem of shortages more acute. Adjusted for the burden of chronic disease, hospital discharge rates are significantly lower than in other OECD countries. The availability of medical technology is skewed towards the private sector, with many high-cost interventions still scarce within the public sector and beyond the reach of most of the population. Furthermore, the introduction of innovative patented medicines has slowed in the public sector due to cost considerations, and there also remain barriers to accepting even cost-effective innovative technologies. Market penetration of generic medicines is also below expectations as compared with developed countries, in spite of the greater benefits such penetration would bring to Mexico. Medical information systems have also lagged behind, although there has been some progress in establishing a system-wide health information platform and the provision of services to the rural poor through telemedicine. The promise of electronic health records (ECE), mobile technology and information platforms directed to patients still has to be realized.

The objective to establish a universal national health system fell short of expectations during the Peña Nieto administration between 2012 and 2018. Per capita public health spending decreased for the first time in decades as a result of small but significant reductions in the funding for the non-insured. Out-of-pocket spending has not reduced significantly, although catastrophic expenditure has remained at the levels set in previous administrations in part through Seguro Popular and in part due to the increase in low-cost private medical consultations and access to generic medicines. Furthermore, coverage by Seguro Popular did not expand significantly to include additional high-cost interventions.

Over the last decade, medical specialty services exchange agreements across public institutions have been in operation to increase efficiency deploying public resources. Though revamped in recent years, their performance remains below what could be achieved through a truly universal programme to provide unfettered access to public hospitals, regardless of institutional coverage. The segmented governance of the health system is perhaps the biggest obstacle to a universal health system, given that social insurance institutions largely operate outside MoH regulation. This situation hinders the development of a stronger regulatory authority capable of addressing barriers to access and quality of care.

Introduction

■ Chapter summary

- Mexico is a federation of 32 state governments including Mexico City, the seat of federal government; it is the 11th most populous country in the world with over 124 million residents.
- The population is relatively young, with just 7% of the population 65 years and older. However, declining mortality rates and fertility rates are contributing to the gradual ageing of the population.
- Poverty and food insecurity are persistent challenges; these disproportionately affect rural residents.
- Diabetes and ischaemic heart disease were the main causes of death in 2015, with diabetes representing a major challenge for disease control.
- Obesity prevalence is second highest in the world (behind the United States), and childhood overweight and obesity is highest globally.

■ 1.1 Geography and sociodemography

Mexico, officially the United Mexican States, is located in the south of North America. Its territory spans a total area of 1 964 375 km², which is divided into a continental area of 1 959 248 km² and an island area of 5127 km²

(Figure 1.1). Geographically, Mexico is the 15th largest country in the world; and the sixth largest in the Americas, behind Canada, the United States of America, Brazil, Greenland and Argentina (CIA, 2016). Mexico has three international borders: the United States to the north (3152 km); the Republic of Guatemala to the south (956 km); and Belize to the southeast (193 km). Mexico's Pacific coastline is 7828 km and 3249 km along the Gulf of Mexico and Caribbean Sea (INEGI, nd, *Extensión territorial*).

As of 2017, Mexico had a total population of over 124 million inhabitants (Table 1.1), placing it as the 11th most populous country in the world. Mexico is made up of a federal government and 31 states (32 including Mexico City). The State of Mexico is the most populous (13.5% of the total population), followed by Mexico City (7.5%) and Jalisco (6.6%). The least populous states are Baja California Sur (0.6%), Colima (0.6%) and Campeche (0.8%) (INEGI, nd, *Indicadores por entidad federativa*). In 2016, 77% of Mexico's population lived in urban areas and the remaining 23% in rural localities. In contrast, in 1960 the urban population was only 51%. It was estimated in 2016 that up to 58% of the rural population lived in poverty, compared with about 39% of the urban population (World Bank, 2018).

Approximately 15 million people identify as Indigenous (about 12% of the total population), and roughly 6.6 million speak an Indigenous language. At least 1.38 million people (1.1% of the total) recognize having African ancestry (INEGI, 2015). Great diversity characterizes Mexico's Indigenous populations: they speak 68 languages and live throughout the country, often in small, isolated communities. Indigenous Peoples compare less favourably to the general population with regard to poverty and health status indicators, although disparities have not been systematically measured. In 2000, the infant mortality rate among the Totonacas, the worse-off Indigenous group, was 57.0 per 1000 liveborn and 37.9 among the Mayans, the best-off Indigenous group, compared with 24.9 in the general population (Zolla, 2007). Among Indigenous language speakers, only 58.3% of married women of fertile age used contraceptives in 2009, compared with 73.5% among non-speakers (Hernández López, Hernández Vázquez & Sánchez Castillo, 2013). A large part of the afrodescendant population maintains a cultural identity, live in close-knit communities in the coastal regions of the states of Guerrero and Oaxaca and in communities in Veracruz and in Coahuila, and are exposed to discrimination and poverty (Velázquez & Iturralde, 2012).

FIG. 1.1 Political division of the country (32 states)

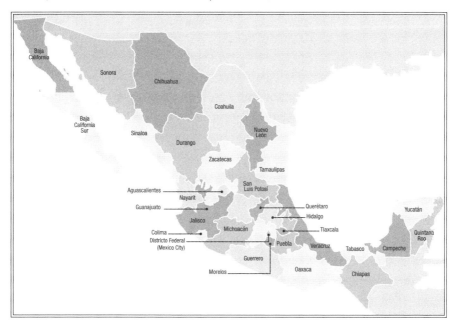

Source: Ciclo escolar (2018)

TABLE 1.1 Population and demographic indicators, 1991–2017

INDICATOR	1991	2000	2005	2010	2015	2017
Total population (per thousand)[a]	85 749	98 785	105 669	113 749	121 348	124 042
Population, women (% of total)	50.56	50.86	51.05	51.06	51.04	51.03
Population from 0 to 14 years (% of total)	38.80	34.25	31.88	29.57	27.58	26.86
Population aged 65 and over (% of total)	4.21	4.98	5.56	6.12	6.76	7.07
Population growth (annual %)[a]	1.84	1.27	1.35	1.42	1.14	1.05
Population density (per km²)	43.65	50.29	53.79	57.91	61.77	63.15
Fertility (children per woman aged 15–49 years)[a]	3.36	2.67	2.47	2.31	2.18	2.13
Crude birth rate (per 1000 inhabitants)[a]	28.20	23.51	21.58	19.96	18.45	17.78
Gross mortality rate (per 1000 inhabitants)[a]	5.11	4.51	4.74	5.30	5.78	5.90
Dependency ratio	75.48	64.55	59.85	55.49	52.32	51.37
Primary school completion[c]	–	86.30	91.80	94.90	98.3	–
Secondary school completion[c]	–	74.90	77.00	83.30	87.7	–
Post-secondary completion[c]	–	57.02	58.25	62.23	64.82	–

[a]CONAPO (2018a), [b]INEGI (2003), [c]Refers to students who finished the level as a proportion of those initiating it (INEGI, 2018b), [d]Nava (2016)

Sources: INEGI, (2018b) Characteristics of households, unless otherwise indicated.

As indicated in Table 1.1, Mexico has a young population, but the population structure is gradually ageing. In 2017, 27% of the population was under 14 years old and 7% were 65 and older. Between 2010 and 2015, 18 states experienced net-positive internal migration, with the State of Mexico receiving the greatest population gain, followed by Nuevo León and Querétaro. Over 1 million people (less than 1% of the population) were born outside of Mexico (INEGI, 2016a). In 2014 about 11.7 million Mexicans lived in the United States and Canada (González Barrera, 2015).

Mexico is vulnerable to natural disasters, including hurricanes that hit both the Atlantic and Pacific coasts and great seismic and volcanic activity due to unstable tectonic plates, with more than 2000 volcanoes concentrated in the south of the country, 14 of which are active (Macías, 2005; Yarza, 2003). Mexico spans the Nearctic and Neotropical climatic regions, with large variations in altitude, from sea level to high plateaus ranging from 1000 metres in the north to 2300 metres in the centre of the country and mountains that reach altitudes of 5700 metres. Mexico is therefore characterized by a wide variety of climates that produce great biodiversity. In the north, arid climates are predominant, while in the south and southeast, climates are hot-humid and sub-humid (INEGI, 2005; Secretaría de Economía, 2016).

1.2 Economic context

Mexico is the 12th largest economy in the world and second largest in Latin American based on its gross domestic product (GDP) as measured in US$ PPP. Mexico is an upper middle-income country with one of the highest per capita incomes in Latin America. Mexico is a member of the OECD, the G20, the Pacific Alliance and the North American Free Trade Agreement (NAFTA), which was replaced with the United States–Mexico–Canada Agreement (USMCA) in 2020.

In 2017, Mexico's GDP amounted to more than US$ 2 344 billion PPP or approximately US$ 18 149 per capita compared with an average of US$ 15 777 in Latin America and the Caribbean, and US$ 43 351 in the OECD. The annual GDP growth rate fell from 4.9% in 2000 to 2.3% in 2005, but rose to 5.1% in 2010. From 2015 to 2017, there was an economic contraction, the end result of a long-term decrease in the industrial growth rate from 2000 to 2017 (Table 1.2).

The benefits of economic growth at the national level have not affected all Mexicans equally. Mexico has the largest income inequality in the OECD. In 2016, the Gini coefficient – which measures inequality within populations between 0 and 1, with 1 being the most unequal – stood at 0.46, as against the OECD average of 0.32 (OECD, 2018f). However, this is still lower than in several other Latin American countries, including Brazil and Colombia (0.51 in 2015), and Guatemala (0.48 in 2014), but is similar in magnitude to Argentina, Ecuador and Peru (World Bank, 2018). The relatively high level of income inequality in Mexico means that the richest 10% of the population earned 20 times more than the poorest 10%.

Mexico's unemployment rate rose from 2.6% in 2000, to 5.3% in 2010 (Table 1.2). The unemployment rate decreased during the 2010s as a result of the government's structural reforms and macroeconomic policies (see section 2.1). In 2017, the unemployment rate was 3.5%, representing a decrease of 2 percentage points over the previous 7 years. Poverty fell in such a way that the population below the poverty line (US$ 3.10 per day) and living in extreme poverty (US$ 1.90 per day) decreased to less than half that observed in 2000. However, poverty levels have remained stable since 2016 (CONEVAL, 2018).

In 2013, the economic participation rate for Mexicans aged 15 to 64 was 60.8%, five points below the OECD average. The economic participation rate in Mexico continues to be higher for men (78.3%) than for women (45%). The average number of hours worked per year in the country was 2237, which was higher than that of the OECD, which reports 1770 hours worked per year. In the same year, Mexico's unemployment rate for people aged 15 and over was 4.9%, below the OECD average of 7.9%. In particular, the unemployment rate among young people between 15 and 24 was 9.5%, below the OECD average of 16% (OECD, 2018c).

The country has implemented a multidimensional approach to assessing poverty based on income and access to social services, such as health services, housing, social security and education, among others. In general, Mexico's multidimensional poverty rate remains high but stable (46.0% of the total population in 2010 compared with 46.2% in 2014), although progress was made in improving social conditions, particularly with regard to access to health care measured as the percentage of the population enjoying financial protection (CONEVAL, 2018).

TABLE 1.2 Macroeconomic indicators for Mexico, 2000–2017

INDICATOR	2000	2005	2010	2015	2017
GDP at current prices (in Mexican pesos, billions)	6694	9563	13 366	18 537	21 767
GDP (in billion US$ PPP)	1098	1342	1743	2170	2344
GDP per capita (Mexican pesos)	65 805	88 158	113 932	147 243	168 523
GDP per capita (US$ PPP)	10 799	12 370	14 859	17 239	18 149
Average annual GDP growth rate (%)	4.9	2.3	5.1	3.3	2.0
Public expenditure (% of GDP)	12.7	—	21.4	21.6	21.0[a]
Value added in industry (% of GDP)	34.2	32.8	32.4	30.0	29.9
Value added in agriculture (% of GDP)	3.3	3.1	3.2	3.2	3.4
Labour force (total, millions)	40.3	44.8	50.5	56.0	58.1
Unemployment, total (% of labour force)	2.6	3.6	5.3	4.3	3.5
Poverty rate (headcount ratio)	45.1	41.0	37.1	—	34.8[a]
Income inequality (Gini coefficient)	0.51	0.49	0.45	—	0.43[a]
Real interest rate	5.2	3.6	0.7	0.7	1.1
Official exchange rate (US$)	9.5	10.9	12.6	—	—

GDP: Gross domestic product; PPP: Power purchasing parity

[a]2016 data

Source: World Bank (2018)

1.3 **Political context**

Mexico is a federal, representative and democratic republic governed by the Constitution of 1917. The federation consists of 32 states, including the government of Mexico City, the seat of federal government. The republic consists of three counter-balancing powers: executive, legislative and judicial, represented at both the federal and state levels.

States are sovereign entities with their own state laws subordinate to a state constitution, which is itself consistent with the federal Constitution. Specific functions within the 32 states are delegated to 2464 municipal governments (or mayoralties in the case of Mexico City), ranging from 570 municipalities in Oaxaca to five each in Baja California and Baja California Sur. State governments elect assemblies of deputies for 3-year terms, which can be renewed for up to two or four terms, depending on each state's constitution. State residents also elect representatives to the federal Congress and Senate. Executive power is vested in the president at the federal level and governors at the state level. Both the national president and the state governors hold office for non-renewable 6-year terms. Municipal presidents are elected every 3 years and can be renewed for one term.

The federal legislature – the Congress – consists of a lower and an upper chamber. The lower Chamber of Deputies is made up of 500 representatives elected for up to four 3-year terms. Of the 500 deputies, 300 are directly elected by residents within electoral districts and 200 are allocated according to proportional representation across five regions in the country. The upper Chamber of Senators – the Senate – is made up of 128 representatives elected for a maximum of two 6-year terms. Two senators are directly elected by residents in each state, with an additional senator elected for the first minority and 32 additional senators elected according to proportional representation. While federal and state-level elected officials had traditionally been restricted to serving for only one term, multiple terms were introduced in 2018 to encourage more effective representation.

All legislative bills need to be approved by both the lower and upper chambers through a simple majority and can be formulated by either chamber or directly through presidential decrees. In practice, most health laws have been introduced by the lower chamber. International treaties have to be approved by the upper. With regard to the health care system, treaties include the WHO Framework Convention on Tobacco Control (2005) and the Pan American Sanitary Code (1929), as well as its Protocol Annex (1954). Constitutional changes need to be approved by a two thirds majority and have to be ratified by a simple majority of state legislative bodies. The members of the Supreme Court of Justice of the Nation are nominated by the president and approved by the Senate without a fixed term period.

Judicial power is exercised in the Supreme Court, in the Federal Electoral Court, in the Collegiate and Unitary Circuit Courts and in the District Courts. The administration and vigilance of judicial powers is controlled by the Council of the Federal Judicature, with the exception of the Supreme Court, whose members are appointed by the Senate for a 15-year term, based on nominations by the president. The Supreme Court is the highest judicial court and constitutional body in Mexico.

From 1917 to 1997, the executive and legislative branches of government were dominated by the Institutional Revolutionary Party (PRI) and its predecessors, after which PRI lost its majority rule in Congress (Casar, 2013). In 2000, PRI lost the federal presidency for the first time in its history, in favour of President Vicente Fox from the National Action Party (PAN). Between 1994 and 2018, no president's party had a majority in Congress, and policies had to be negotiated across party lines. Between 2000 and 2018, Congress approved just 81% to 89% of the presidents' initiatives, finally acting as a check and balance on the executive branch.

Given PRI's continuity since 1917 and its dominance in Congress, the executive branch was the most important position of power in the country, with Congress rubber-stamping most executive initiatives. Until 1989, state governors were mostly imposed through PRI's party machinery, when PRI lost its first governorship since 1917 to an incoming PAN candidate. PRI held power through a corporatist political representation structure, with three main sectors nominating representatives to Congress: industrial workers, peasants and the popular sector, while industrialists and merchants influenced government through official, obligatory representation associations. Official trade unions and organizations arranged each sector in a pyramidal structure cemented through clientelist politics (Córdova, 1972). However, beginning in 1988, President Carlos Salinas de Gortari privatized most of the parastatal sector and reduced the size of state governments, which initiated a period of what came to be perceived as neoliberal rule. This period was characterized by the downgrading of the power of corporatist organizations. Political reform led to an expansion in the number of political parties, going beyond PRI and the loyal opposition of PAN and fringe left-wing parties.

Mexico had nine political parties registered at the federal level as of 2018. Besides PRI, three other parties were major contenders in the most recent federal elections: the right-of-centre PAN, the left-of-centre Partido de la Revolución Democrática (PRD) and the newly established Movement for National Regeneration party (Morena). This latter party was single-handedly established as a new force by ex-PRI politician Andrés Manuel López Obrador, who drew support from dissident members of other leftist parties but also from PRI and PAN. Elections in July 2018 delivered an upset to traditional party dominance, with Morena winning the presidency on an anticorruption platform by a landslide 53% of the vote. Morena also gained the absolute majority in both chambers of Congress. PAN obtained 22% of the presidential vote – an historically low result – and PRI received only 16% of electoral support. It is expected that Morena will have ample powers to introduce sweeping changes in Congress. Furthermore, Morena also has the majority in most of the state assemblies, in addition to having won five of the nine governorships that held elections in 2018. Morena thus has political power to introduce major changes in policy, although changes to the Constitution still require negotiations with opposition parties.

Administrative decentralization starting in the mid-80s and political opposition in Congress since 1997 have transferred greater powers to Congress and the state level, particularly for health policy and health services administration. However, these decentralizing reforms have been contaminated by clientelist politics and corruption at the state level, while weak nongovernmental organizations (NGOs) among professional associations have failed to act as a countervailing force against the federal government's power. Corruption continues to plague Mexican politics and governance: in 2017, the country was ranked 135th out of 180 countries on corruption as measured by Transparency International, a slight improvement over earlier years (Transparency International, 2018).

1.4 **Health status**

1.4.1 *Life expectancy*

Life expectancy at birth in Mexico has improved dramatically: from 34 years in 1930 to 75 in 2017. Life expectancy has increased at a faster rate than in other industrialized countries, but with a significant delay. According to OECD statistics, Canada reached Mexico's current life expectancy in 1979, while the United States attained it in 1989. The life expectancy gap with respect to Canada is currently 6.9 years and with the United States, 3.4 years. Among OECD countries, Mexico's life expectancy is above only those of Latvia and Lithuania (OECD, 2018d).

Women in Mexico live on average to 77.7 years of age, and men to 72. The difference in life expectancy between the sexes has remained relatively constant in recent years, between 4.0 and 4.8 years from 1960 to 2016; a smaller gap than in Japan (6.2 years). The differences in life expectancy across Mexico's 32 states have decreased, from 8.8 years in 1970 between states with the lowest and highest life expectancy, to a difference of 3.4 years in 2017. In the last 10 years, both sexes in Mexico City have had the longest life expectancies in the country while residents in the state of Guerrero, among the poorest in the country, have had the shortest.

Following the Mexican Revolution in 1910, the country experienced very high population growth, reaching a peak annual growth rate of 3.5% in the 1970s. Over this time, Mexico's population has doubled every 20 years (Ordorica, 2014). This situation was recognized as a serious challenge to economic and social development and triggered vigorous family planning approaches as government policy. Today, the population is growing at almost 1% per annum, with a national fertility rate in 2015 at 2.3 children per woman (INEGI, 2016a). Mexico's population is projected to start decreasing after 2050.

TABLE 1.3 Mortality and health indicators for Mexico, 1990–2017

INDICATOR	1990	2000	2005	2010	2015	2017
Life expectancy at birth[a]	70.93	74.73	75.22	74.75	74.71	74.88
Life expectancy at birth, women[a]	73.94	77.41	77.8	77.89	77.56	77.75
Life expectancy at birth, men[a]	67.97	72.04	72.62	71.64	71.85	72.03
Mortality rate, adults, women[b]	118.96	93.23	88.82	84.83	79.74	78.00
Mortality rate, adults, males[c]	212.19	166.09	158.10	150.52	141.94	138.00
Infant mortality per 1000 live births	34.91	22.55	18.28	16.15	14.21	13.71

[a]Years. [b] For every 1000 adult women. [c] For every 1000 adult men
Sources: CONAPO (2018a), Banco Mundial (2018a; 2018b)

The level of social development varies considerably across states. The 2012 Human Development Index (HDI) report assessing life expectancy, education and income, identified Mexico City as having the country's highest HDI (0.83), while the states of Guerrero and Chiapas occupied the last places (0.68 and 0.67 respectively); the national average was 0.75.

■ **1.4.2** *Mortality*

Mexico's all-cause mortality rate has decreased in recent years, although the mortality rate for men is considerably higher than for women (Table 1.3). Women's mortality rates decreased from 119 deaths per 1000 in 1990, to 78 in 2017; during that same time men's rates decreased from 212 per 1000 in 1990, to 138 in 2017. A decrease of 66% was maintained over time for both groups, despite the absolute differences. The infant mortality rate (IMR) has also decreased considerably. Although Mexico continues to have one of the highest IMRs in the Americas, it is lower than the Latin American and Caribbean average, which was 15 deaths per 1000 live births in 2017 (World Bank, 2018). While differences in mortality across states with the highest and lowest HDI have been markedly reduced, maternal mortality is still seven times higher in the poorest state compared with the richest (Observatorio de Mortalidad Materna, 2018). Infant mortality rates also show important differences across the richest and poorest states and municipalities in Mexico, with a rate of 12.9 and 3.0 deaths per 1000 births in Mexico City and in one of its richest municipalities, Benito Juárez, compared with 24.4 deaths per 1000 births in Guerrero and 60.8 in Cochoapa el Grande, one of its poorest municipalities (CONAPO, 2005).

The crude death rate has decreased slowly despite the increased longevity of older adults. A recent epidemiological transition in Mexico has seen the burden of disease shift from communicable to noncommunicable diseases. According to a Global Burden of Disease study (IHME, 2018), in 1990, 44% of the total burden of disease was from chronic disease, rising to 78% in 2016. In 2015, diabetes was the leading cause of death in men and women, followed by heart disease (see Table 1.4). The study identified that in 2013 the 10 leading causes of years of life lost due to premature death (YLPD) corresponded to: 1) ischaemic heart disease, 2) chronic kidney disease, 3) diabetes, 4) traffic accidents, 5) interpersonal violence, 6) congenital anomalies, 7) lower respiratory infections, 8) cerebrovascular diseases, 9) complications of premature birth and 10) cirrhosis due to alcohol. Between 1990 and 2013, chronic kidney disease as a factor in YLPD increased by 241%, while diabetes and ischaemic heart disease increased by 32% and 38%, respectively. According to the US Chamber of Commerce, chronic diseases in Mexico account for productivity losses equivalent to

5.3% of GDP. Diabetes and chronic kidney disease were estimated to cost the social insurance scheme for private sector employees (IMSS) nearly 11% of its health budget, representing 0.25% of Mexico's GDP (Figueroa Lara, González Block & Alarcón Irigoyen, 2016).

Mortality from infectious diseases decreased significantly since 1990, although deaths associated with conditions such as lower respiratory infections and acute diarrhoeal disease remain the two most common causes of death in children under five (Table 1.4). The mortality rate for diabetes mellitus between 1990 to 2015 rose from 30.6 to 81.1 per 1000 total deaths, representing a dramatic increase. Similarly, the mortality rate due to ischaemic heart diseases increased from 35.2 in 1990 to 72.5 in 2015.

TABLE 1.4 Mortality rates in Mexico by selected causes, 1990–2015

INDICATOR	1990	2000	2005	2010	2015
Diabetes mellitus	30.57	47.1	63.49	72.88	81.13
Ischaemic heart disease	35.17	44.29	50.33	62.16	72.45
Homicide (men)	30.92	19.32	16.63	41.83	30.78
Prostate cancer (45 years and over)	18.42	21.71	22.47	21.5	21.33
Motor vehicle traffic accidents (men)	20	16.82	20.27	20.68	19.23
Arterial hypertension	8.08	9.87	12.19	15.54	19.15
Breast cancer (women)	12.86	14.52	15.55	16.36	18.1
Children under 5 years old by LRI	123.12	46.58	33.95	22.83	16.45
Suicides (per 100 000 inhabitants)	2.4	3.4[a]	—	4.6	5.1[a]
Youth suicide mortality rate	5.49	8.88	10.76	11.99	14.84
Cervical cancer	11.8	9.99	12.29	12.66	11.75
Children under 5 years old by ADD	24.91	19.48	15.74	12.84	11.57
Motor vehicle traffic accidents (women)	144.3	30.11	21.2	8.99	7.26
HIV /AIDS	3.79	3.44	4.63	4.79	4.24
Pulmonary tuberculosis	3.56	2.55	2.4	4.16	3.85

ADD: acute diarrhoeal disease; LRI: Lower respiratory infections

[a] Rate for 1999 and 2016, respectively

Notes: Rates per 1000 deaths unless otherwise noted.

Source: CONAPO (2018b)

Mexico is close to the global average in mortality rates for ischaemic heart diseases and heart attack, which are the leading causes of death in the majority of higher-income countries. However, Mexico's mortality rates from these causes are higher than in OECD countries that have undergone more advanced epidemiological and demographic transitions.

The death rate due to homicide in 1990 is close to that reported in 2015 and remains the third leading cause of death among men. High homicides rates remerged in the last 10 years or so mainly due to a growing illicit drug trade problem, concentrated in a few Mexican states. While significant reductions have been observed in women's mortality rates associated with traffic accidents, deaths from motor vehicle traffic accidents remain the fifth leading cause of death for men. The mortality rate associated with suicide maintains an upward trend, particularly among youth. The registered suicide rate increased from 2.4 suicides per 100 thousand inhabitants in 1990 to 3.4 in 1999 and 4.6 in 2010 (Jiménez-Ornelas & Cardiel-Téllez, 2013), while for 2017 it was 5.2 (INEGI, 2019). Among youth, the trend increased from 5.49 per 1000 deaths in 1990 to 14.84 in 2015 (Table 1.4).

1.4.3 *Morbidity*

The emphasis on influencing healthy lifestyles is becoming more prevalent given the increasing burden of disability and premature death caused by chronic diseases. In Mexico, the economic burden of diabetes mellitus was more than 360 billion pesos (US$ 18.6 billion) in 2013, equivalent to 2.25% of its GDP (Barraza Lloréns, 2015). Globally, Mexico ranks second after the United States in obesity prevalence (OECD, 2018c). Today, at least one in three Mexicans is obese, increasing from 23.7% in 2000 to 33.3% in 2016 (Gutiérrez et al., 2012). More worrying is the fact that Mexico ranks first in the world in the prevalence of childhood overweight and obesity combined. In the case of preschool children (under 5 years old), prevalence of overweight and obesity was 9.7% in 2012; while for the school-age children (5 to 11 years old) it was 34.4%. From 1999 to 2006 the combined prevalence of overweight and obesity in school-age children rose from 26.9% to 34.8% and remained unchanged from 2006 to 2012. Physical activity indicators show that 22.7% of adolescents are inactive and 18.3% are moderately active.

In the group aged 19 to 69 years, this indicator corresponded to 17.4% and 11.9%, respectively.

The costs of diabetes care and its burden on public institutions and consumers were estimated by Barraza et al. (2015) at 1.1% of GDP in 2013, with diabetes complications representing 87.2% of the total diabetes expenditure. The costliest complication is the most advanced stage of nephropathy (E5), accounting for 38.2% of the total expenditure, followed by acute myocardial infarction (AMI) at 17.9%. The IMSS allocates 11% of its health budget to diabetes, which is 38% of the total national diabetes expenditure by all public institutions.

Progress has been made to reduce the prevalence of risk factors affecting health (Table 1.5). However, 28.2% of Mexican households continue to experience food insecurity, suggesting that lack of income is an important social determinant of health. Low weight, short stature, wasting and underweight in children under 5 years old have decreased from 1988 to 2012; however, the prevalence of acute malnutrition has remained relatively constant since 1999. The national prevalence of anaemia in preschool children was 23.3% in 2012, with the highest prevalence seen in children 12 to 23 months of age; in school-aged children this was 10.1%. Between 1999 and 2012, the prevalence of anaemia in school-aged children decreased by 5 percentage points.

Between 2005 and 2017, there was a reduction in cigarette consumption, fatal traffic accidents under the influence of alcohol and deaths in work-related accidents (Table 1.5). In 2015, while the consumption of alcohol per capita (4.8 litres) was lower than the European Union average, alcohol cirrhosis was the 10th main cause of YLPD. Although the proportion of regular daily smokers with respect to the total population (7.6%) remained constant from 2009 to 2015, the prevalence of smoking in Mexico is lower than in other OECD countries as well as compared with other middle-income countries such as India, China, the Russian Federation and Indonesia (OECD, 2018c). However, the incidence of chronic obstructive pulmonary disease (COPD) ranks 10 on the list of the main causes of YLPD adjusted for disability.

Mental health is also a challenge in Mexico. In 2003, up to 28% of the population presented with at least one mental health disorder included in the International Classification of Mental Illnesses during their lifetime; 13% reported it in the last 12 months and 5.8% in the last 30 days (Medina-Mora,

2003). The National Survey of Mental Health recorded that 18% of the urban population of working age (15–64 years of age) suffer from a mood disorder such as anxiety, depression or phobia, while 3 million people are addicted to alcohol, 13 million are smokers and there are more than 400 thousand addicts to psychotropics (Medina-Mora et al., 2007).

TABLE 1.5 Risk factors related to health in Mexico, 2005 or earliest year and 2017 or latest year

INDICATOR	2005	2017
Amount of fruits and vegetables available (kg/person/year) (1)	172.06	163.31[a]
Proportion of obesity (BMI> 30) (%) (2)	23.7[c]	33.3[c]
Consumption of alcohol per capita (litres of alcohol in the population aged 15 to 65) (3)	—	4.8[c]
Fatal traffic accidents under the influence of alcohol (4)	473	297[c]
Consumption of tobacco per capita in daily smokers (cigarettes per day) (5)	9.4[d]	7.7[e]
Proportion of regular daily smokers in the population aged 15 and over (%) (5)	7.6[d]	7.6[e]
Occupational diseases (total) (6)	7292	14 159
Occupational accidents (total) (6)	295 594	410 266
Deaths in work-related accidents (total) (6)	1112	993

[a]Data for 2013. [b]Data for 2000. [c]Data for 2016. [d]Data for 2009. [e]Data for 2015

Sources: (1) FAO (2017), (2) INSP (2018a), (3) Villatoro Velázquez et al. (2017); (4) INEGI (2017), (5) OPS (2017), (6) STPS (2018)

Table 1.6 shows a mixed picture with regards to morbidity. Acute respiratory infections, chickenpox, hepatitis A, intestinal infections and other helminthiasis have decreased, while problems related to conjunctivitis and gingivitis have increased. While AIDS cases have remained stable, diagnoses of asymptomatic HIV and new HIV cases have increased. This suggests that while the AIDS epidemic is under control, avoidable infections are not being averted as far as possible. Other problems such as urinary tract infections, ulcers, acute otitis, asthma, pneumonia and bronchopneumonia and respiratory tuberculosis have maintained a steady rate.

TABLE 1.6 Selected disease morbidity rates in Mexico, 2005 and 2017

INDICATOR	2005	2017
Acute respiratory infections	25 013	21 346
Intestinal infections	4476	4672
Urinary tract infection	2988	3622
Ulcers, gastritis and duodenitis	1346	1231
Conjunctivitis	250.5	1155
Vulvovaginitis[a]	—	1005.4
Gingivitis and periodontal disease	422.5	947.8
Acute otitis media	709	687.6
Obesity	—	559.8
Hypertension[b]	487.8	547.5
Type 2 diabetes[c]	373.3	405.1
Hyperplasia of the prostate[d]	—	336.21
Asthma	272.62	213.1
Chickenpox	306.1	124.3
Other helminthiasis	376.5	118.1
Pneumonia and bronchopneumonia	161.7	105.1
Respiratory tuberculosis	14.3	13.8
Asymptomatic HIV infection	3.8	6.6
New cases diagnosed with HIV[e]	—	8114
Hepatitis A	20.09	5.44
AIDS	4.11	4.53
Hepatitis B	0.59	0.48

[a]Incidence per 100 000 female inhabitants, [b]Incidence per 100 000 inhabitants over 14 years, [c]Incidence per 100 000 inhabitants over 10 years, [d]Incidence per 100 000 male inhabitants over 25 years, [e]Centro Nacional para la Prevención y Control del VIH y el sida (2018)

Note: Incidence per 100 000 inhabitants unless otherwise indicated

Source: DGE (2018) unless otherwise stated

2

Organization and governance

■ Chapter summary

- The Mexican health system evolved from mandatory employer-based private insurance, worker protection and campaigns to control infectious disease epidemics in the beginning of the 20th century.
- Article 4 of the Constitution has guaranteed the right to health protection since 1983, while Article 1 recognizes the human rights – including health – declared by the International Covenant on Economic, Social and Cultural rights.
- The health system provides little choice to consumers, and patient rights are weakly overseen in practice.
- Health coverage is achieved through a mix of social insurance schemes, a voluntary public programme for the uninsured, and private insurance, which collectively cover about 85% of the Mexican population.
- The social insurance system is dominated by two national institutions covering formal sector salaried employees and funded by the federal government, employers and employees: IMSS for private sector employees (33% of the population) and ISSSTE (7.4% of the population). Other federal-level schemes cover the army and navy, while state-based schemes cover state bureaucrats.

- Seguro Popular – the voluntary coverage programme funded by the federal and state governments, and with some funding by enrollees above the poverty line – covered 43.5% of the population with a limited benefits package in 2015.
- The federal and state governments act as payers, providers and regulators of health services while the social insurance institutions integrate these functions through vertically structured organizations.
- Covered individuals have access only to the providers and facilities employed by those vertical organizations; thus, there is no choice of provider, unless they pay out-of-pocket for services outside of their provider networks.
- Social insurance institutions, and to a large extent state schemes, own their health infrastructure and hire salaried employees, who are mostly unionized through institutional trade unions.
- The Ministry of Health oversees a health information system through a coordinated set of resource, service and performance indicators.

■ 2.1 **Historical background**

■ **2.1.1** *Formation of the health system*

The Mexican health system evolved with the industrialization of the post-colonial agrarian society and the development of the federation. Its history can be understood as the interplay of four broad trends. The first was the development of accident indemnity organized by employers through private health insurance that was intended as a response to the health and social risks emerging alongside industrialization at the beginning of the 20th century. The second is the political subordination of worker and entrepreneur organizations to the federal government by the late 1920s and the culmination of this process in the 1940s through the establishment of the IMSS. The third, starting in the late 19th century and consolidated in the 1917 Constitution was the response by the federal government to epidemics threatening urban areas as well as military and agro-industrial enclaves in the Gulf of Mexico. The fourth trend was the federal government's response to the health care needs of the rural masses and the urban poor through social assistance. It can also be mentioned in this context the participation of the private sector in addressing the health needs of more affluent city dwellers from the 1940s as contributing to the slow roll out of IMSS at least until the 1960s (González Block, 1990; 2018).

The health needs of a rising urban middle class and the development of a French-influenced medical profession led to the establishment of a number of professional and regulatory institutions from the middle of the 19th century. Foremost was the National Academy of Medicine, which contributed to the professionalization of medicine in the country, while the General Health Council oversaw epidemic control and introduced modern public health. At the turn of the century the governors of the more industrial states in central and northern Mexico introduced statutes of limitations for employers and indemnity against work-related accidents as an inalienable right, measures that followed the example of European Christian Democratic and Liberal political movements. Federal government legislation also established the medical profession's monopoly in arbitrating complaints and in caring for those harmed in industrial accidents and by occupational diseases. Indemnity legislation encouraged entrepreneurs to seek private insurance and strengthened the autonomous organizations of workers.

The failed succession of the dictator Porfirio Díaz in 1911, triggered the Mexican Revolution and years of civil war. In this context, a few states under the leadership of revolutionary strongmen introduced legislation seeking collaboration between the nascent proletariat and the capitalist class. In 1915, the governor of the state of Jalisco instituted a social fund resembling those legislated in Germany by Bismarck in 1883. In the same year, Governor Salvador Alvarado of Yucatán state mandated funds to address accident prevention and indemnity, and protected working children and pregnant women from extreme forms of exploitation practised in the production of sisal, a leading export crop.

Also in 1915, the Revolution's strongmen, Venustiano Carranza and Álvaro Obregón, took over Mexico City and mobilized the urban proletariat against their rivals, Emiliano Zapata and Francisco Villa, who refused to accept their rule. While this shift in authority initially empowered urban workers, they were eventually repressed by the government and subordinated through politically loyal, official organizations. Relative peace was achieved by the strongmen through the promulgation of the 1917 Constitution, which instituted the modern electoral process.

The 1917 Constitution formalized the country's health system, with important amendments in 1929 and 1983. Article 123 legislated labour rights, including the right to accident indemnity and protection against occupational risks, the protection of women and children, and the promotion of social insurance funds. Labour law was delegated as a responsibility of sovereign state legislatures, most of whom proceeded to enact local laws focusing exclusively on accident indemnity protections. The 1917 Constitution also established the federal government's responsibility for so-called General Health, primarily for epidemic control, leading to the establishment of the Department of Health. Article 5 established the legal legitimacy of the liberal professions, protecting the private practice of medicine and the recognition of professional colleges (González Block, 1990).

■ **2.1.2** *The rise of public health*

President Obregón (1920–1924) established the Department of Health and started building modern facilities and laboratories with the aim of addressing the dire health situation left after the Revolution. Obregón gave special priority to the eradication of yellow fever from the ports in the Gulf of Mexico, which threatened the movement of troops and the development of agro-industry and oil production as well as international commerce. This effort also responded to the request by the United States government to work with Mexico towards the elimination of yellow fever from the Gulf area as a whole, including their own important ports such as New Orleans. The United States provided strong incentives and facilitators for these efforts, conditioning the recognition of the newly established revolutionary regime, with the support of the Rockefeller Foundation. The focus was on the implementation of vertical health and sanitation campaigns in the most important urban areas as well as in the training of Mexico's modern public health professionals. The School of Public Health of Mexico was established in 1922, charged with training cadres of public health leaders in the decades to come. Funded by the Rockefeller Foundation, top-level public health officers were trained in the schools of public health at Johns Hopkins and Harvard.

■ **2.1.3** *Development of social insurance institutions*

President Obregón proposed a federal law towards the establishment of workers' compensation, aiming to expropriate and control the funding and management of accident indemnity from employers. The law failed to be passed by Congress partly due to the opposition of employers and state governors, who were reluctant to forgo their executive and legislative control over occupational health, which the Constitution clearly gave them. However, this effort established an important precedent that was to be pursued later. Subsequently, President Plutarco E Calles (1924–1928) proposed a likewise unsuccessful constitutional amendment to enable the federal government to take over social insurance, together with the establishment of a National Institute of Social Insurance (INSS) that was to be funded by employers and the government. The INSS would be governed through a corporatist executive directorate with equal representation from employers, employees and the government, and would be responsible for the provision of health services through its own proprietary infrastructure. Though out of office by 1928, Calles assumed a powerful role as a strongman until 1936, through the so-called *Maximato* period.

The Constitution was amended in 1929 by President Emilio Portes Gil, enabling Congress to enact laws to federalize labour relations – including with respect to occupational health and safety. While the Federal Labour Law was enacted in 1931 by President Pascual Ortiz Rubio (1930–1932), social insurance legislation was not changed, leaving intact the rights and administrative procedures extant at the state level. Even though Mexico joined the International Labour Organization (ILO) in 1931 and federal social insurance legislation had been prepared, employer opposition averted its consideration by Congress, for fear of a negative economic impact in the economy at the time of the Great Depression. In this context, Calles and the ruling party left the establishment of the INSS for the next administration.

The federal government's health policy efforts in the early 1930s focused on establishing coordination agreements with states to strengthen public health campaigns and epidemic control, with continued collaboration and funding by the Rockefeller Foundation. The model was to develop state and municipal capabilities around local health departments following a public health model that had been very successful in the United States. Personal health services were not addressed, as these were considered as the realm either of workers' protection legislation or of the private market.

President Cardenas (1934–1940) focused for the first time on agrarian reform – the chief promise of the Mexican Revolution – and embarked on delivering the peasants from exploitation through the expropriation of large landholdings and the organization of peasant cooperatives, as well as through the modernization of production and credit. His regime was characterized by a high degree of worker mobilization and strikes and was fiercely criticized by Calles during the latter's de facto *Maximato* rule. Cardenas responded by consolidating his power and exiled Calles in 1936, abandoning the plan to establish the INSS and focusing instead on alternative measures in support of agrarian reform, such as supporting medical care for peasants organized under economic collectives. Nonetheless, Cardenas later proposed an alternative scheme for urban social insurance.

The development of health policy in support of agrarian reform resulted from the demand by collectivized peasants for medical care both to recover from illness and to justify absenteeism and the consequent risk of losing their proprietary rights. Private physicians were contracted by collectives while the Department of Health introduced preventive health programmes, thus combining, for the first time, personal health services and public health campaigns under integrated, locally based organizations. Health care funding for these efforts was eventually taken over by the public bank, which provided credit to the collectives in an effort to bolster productivity and credit repayment.

With the ILO's help, Cardenas proposed an urban social insurance scheme aimed at providing health insurance and social benefits to industrial workers through a Social Services Institute (ISS). This institution contrasted sharply with Calles' proposed INSS in that now both public and private providers would participate based on market conditions, while employer, employee and federal funding would be complemented by state government funding to better tailor these social insurance schemes to local conditions. Governance of ISS would not follow the corporatist arrangements proposed for INSS; instead, decision-making would be restricted to a professional board, with workers and employers participating in a consultative as opposed to decision-making capacity. However, ISS was not implemented, coming late in Cardenas' presidency at a time when he was facing opposition to the nationalization of the Mexican oil industry enacted through his oil expropriation decree in March 1938, as well as against further land reform. In this context, the ruling party redesigned the establishment of the INSS into a 6-year plan to be carried out by Cardenas' successor.

2.1.4 *Creation of IMSS and the segmented public health system*

President Cardenas was succeeded in 1940 by President Manuel Avila Camacho (1940–1946) through a highly contested and fraudulent election amidst localized uprisings. In the middle of the Second World War, Camacho prioritized national unity and in June 1941 established a technical commission with ILO's support to formulate the fine details of INSS and to prepare its implementation. At precisely the same time, the United Kingdom commissioned what came to be known as the Beveridge Report, aiming to redress the fragmentation of worker rights and benefits through universal health coverage. A couple of months later – in August 1941 – the United Kingdom and the United States signed the Atlantic Charter, calling for social security based on the report's recommendations and other strategies towards world peace. Early drafts of the report were circulated worldwide by December 1941 and were quickly adopted as a framework to promote solidarity within Allied nations against the Axis powers (Abel-Smith, 1992). In May 1942, Mexico declared war against the Axis powers and became a signatory to the Atlantic Charter. The Charter, and particularly its call for social security, became an instrument of propaganda to support the home front and to instigate the surrendering of enemy soldiers under the prospect of improved life conditions. In Latin American countries, social security was promoted to discourage support towards Nazism and to instil national unity.

An INSS Technical Commission recommended the enactment of social insurance following exactly the model formulated by Calles. In December 1942, Congress promulgated the Social Insurance Law, leading to the establishment of IMSS, substituting "Mexican" for "National" in the institute's title.

Initially, IMSS was to cover 11.6% of the economically active population by 1943, with a broad range of benefits such as pensions, disability insurance and maternity leave. Beneficiaries were mostly salaried private sector employees with permanent contracts in mining, industry, transportation and some service-sector workers (González Block, 2018). The peasantry, which constituted 65.4% of the economically active population as well as most workers in commerce, were excluded, although the Social Insurance Law promised future coverage under special regimes.

Despite the formal participation of officially aligned employer and employee representatives in the formulation process, key employers affected by these reforms, as well as employees at the grass roots, protested against the law just prior to its promulgation and particularly during its rolling out in January 1943. Insurance agencies opposed the expropriation of the workers' compensation business while bankers and other industrialists opposed the imminent expropriation of the health service infrastructure they had developed for their workers. They were also concerned about the disruption of labour relations due to the changes in contract clauses. Workers protested in Mexico City against the threat of losing their benefits, particularly those in key industries such as textiles and newspapers. Physicians also resisted becoming salaried employees of IMSS and the loss of their status as independent liberal professionals. In response to their being excluded from the decision-making process, IMSS medical employees went on strike and demanded a liberal regime for medical practice.

The government addressed protests in the short-term through a mix of co-option and repression. IMSS committed to providing medical services at standards above those offered to employees in the market, rejecting the collaboration of private providers as well as of the new public hospitals that were emerging. This, in turn, divided key medical figures within government, who felt disenfranchised. IMSS physician employees were offered generous salaries well above industry standards, while industrialist protests were quelled through a gradual roll out, which delayed implementation in states outside Mexico City with strong employer-based health infrastructure.

In parallel to the establishment of IMSS, the government merged the Department of Health and the Ministry of Assistance to create the Ministry of Health and Assistance (SSA). The move was partly a response to the concerns of public officials and influential physicians whose institutes and hospitals had been excluded from social insurance funding. Two tertiary care hospitals – the National Cardiology Institute and the Children's

Hospital – were opened and agreements were strengthened with state governments to provide health care for the uninsured and the poor. These arrangements thus established the roots of Mexico's segmented public health system.

In the years to come, IMSS would offer selective health service management rights to those industrialists that were able to keep their infrastructure such as banks and the powerful iron and beer industries in the industrialized state of Nuevo León and its capital Monterrey. In an effort to maintain a firm grip on the labour movement and to stifle potential protest, the government strengthened the exclusive right of IMSS to provide services in all other instances.

2.1.5 *Development of IMSS*

IMSS was implemented very slowly, with only 14.9% of the target population attaining coverage by the end of Avila Camacho's regime in 1946, a total of 3.4% of the economically active population. Implementation was even slower under the presidency of Miguel Alemán (1946–1952), attaining 20.8% of its mandated coverage. This delayed implementation was a result of IMSS needing to invest in its own health care infrastructure.

The model of industrialization based on import-substitution fuelled economic growth after the war, leading to massive rural migration to urban areas and the relative growth of the industrial sector. Following this trend, IMSS coverage picked up under president Adolfo Ruiz Cortínez (1952–1958), yet it reached only one third of its potential coverage or 8.4% of the economically active population. By then Mexico's import-substitution model was beginning to falter. President Adolfo López Mateos (1958–1964) addressed protests stemming from increasingly unequal social rights across critical population groups. López Mateos decreed that IMSS would cover agricultural casual workers, although only during the few months when they were employed on a salaried basis, and excluding sick leave compensation while limiting the amounts paid for accident compensation below the levels set for industrial workers. In 1959, López Mateos also integrated the various federal workers' social insurance schemes under a single institution, creating the Institute for Social Security and Services for State Employees (ISSSTE).

■ 2.1.6 *Deepening of segmentation*

Pro-democracy protests intensified under the presidency of Gustavo Díaz Ordaz (1966–1970), leading to the 1968 student uprising that was violently repressed. In the midst of this crisis, President Luis Echeverría Álvarez (1970–1976) came to power and promised to address inequity, vowing to increase social insurance coverage by 50%. Echeverría decreed a new Social Insurance Law entitling all occupational groups to be gradually covered within differentiated schemes according to their needs and their capacity to contribute. As part of this law, the government initiated the National Programme of Solidarity through Community Cooperation, implemented through the government supply company, the National Company for Subsidies for the Population (CONASUPO), and tasked with providing peasants and small farmers with access to basic medical care through primary medical units and rural hospitals. The programme barred access to IMSS primary care, general and specialty hospitals and excluded workers' compensation and pension benefits.

Funding for the programme was secured mostly from IMSS contributions by increasing the contribution ceilings of high-income employees. While these contributions were in part compensated with additional benefits for the better off, the measure was vigorously opposed by IMSS governors, who cited financial imbalance. Given the opposition, by 1976 IMSS-CONASUPO managed to construct only 200 primary medical units and to cover just a tiny fraction of the uninsured peasantry. In spite of his ambitious Social Insurance Law, Echeverría failed to extend social insurance coverage to any new occupational groups. However, the pressure to redress poverty continued to mount and President José López Portillo (1976–1982) continued to see IMSS as the bulwark against poverty. He sought to surmount financial opposition to its role by expanding its coverage of services through resources coming from the oil boom of the 1980s. The task of extending IMSS services – again through a separate infrastructure – was taken away from CONASUPO and given to the newly established General Coordination of the National Plan for Depressed Zones and Marginalized Groups (COPLAMAR), a bureaucratic agency mandated to fight against poverty. Rather than target poor occupational groups, IMSS-COPLAMAR identified the poor using a set of "social marginalization" indicators, which for the first time enabled the targeting of Indigenous groups and the extreme poor in both urban and rural areas. IMSS-COPLAMAR was able to build close to 3000 medical units and 40 rural hospitals within 2 years, today (under a new organizational form: IMSS-Bienestar) covering close to 12 million people.

While health care coverage was dramatically expanded under López Portillo, this was done at the expense of clarity with respect to whether SSA or IMSS was ultimately responsible for protecting the uninsured, which in turn contributed to government inefficiency. With a faltering economy that was to lead to a deep economic crisis in the 1980s, López Portillo established a Health Coordination Unit to improve efficiency. This led to the recommendation to integrate the diverse, highly fragmented federal health programmes, such as IMSS-COPLAMAR, the Malaria Eradication Programme and the federal hospital system, within state authorities under new, decentralized state ministries of health. The SSA was to retain only specialty hospitals and the National Institutes of Health, with the mandate to focus on governance and set aside the operation of health services.

■   **2.1.7** *Health services decentralization*

President Miguel de la Madrid (1982–1988) implemented the recommendations issued by the Health Coordination Unit in the previous administration, integrating health services at the state level. To support efforts towards a more integrated health system, de la Madrid also sought to promote greater equity with the reform of Article 4 of the Constitution, which established the right to health protection. However, the amendment did not impact Article 123, which covers the rights to health service provision and compensation tied to labour relations, and in so doing established Mexico's segmented sets of health care rights. Article 4 was limited to the federal government's remit for General Health as established by Article 73, which since 1917 had focused on epidemic control and sanitary protection. President de la Madrid addressed the coordination of the segmented government health institutions by decreeing a General Health Law in 1983. The General Health Law legislated the right to health protection within the remit of General Health, a legal figure that explicitly excluded regulation of social insurance institutions by the Ministry of Health, thus curtailing its capacity to mandate the right to health. Instead, the General

Health Law established the notion of a "National Health System" to be coordinated by the MoH and to include all public and private health providers according to their own laws and institutions.

The MoH proceeded to establish decentralized state ministries of health, starting with pilot initiatives in 12 states and aimed to complete the process in all 31 states and the Federal District (now Mexico City) by 1988. Federal hospitals, health centres and IMSS-COPLAMAR units were now organized within state government health facilities under autonomous administrative bodies governed jointly by state and federal governments. IMSS-COPLAMAR units were transferred to these new bodies and fully integrated into state networks. Funding for human resources was transferred through federal funds to the states, equalizing pay across IMSS-COPLAMAR and MoH workforces. While human resources were managed by state ministries of health, national trade unions were kept intact. A National Health Council was established as a policy-making and coordinating body chaired by the federal minister of health, with meetings every 3 months hosted by one of the state ministries of health. State Health Councils were also established to coordinate public and private health providers under state health systems.

IMSS complied reluctantly with this decentralizing mandate during the pilot phase, and transferred medical staff within the IMSS-COPLAMAR programme, yet failed to enact the necessary agreements to transfer medical residents, leading to staff shortages in the hospitals affected. Some state ministries of health failed to promptly address the problem, giving IMSS's director the opportunity to mount a widespread protest against decentralization and calling on the president to suspend it. The president ordered an evaluation, leading to the exoneration of the MoH with respect to how the decentralization process was implemented. However, the evaluation led to time being lost while the economy plummeted in a deep recession. In this context, the Ministry was forced to suspend decentralization indefinitely while maintaining the integration of the health services infrastructure for the non-insured in the initially piloted 12 decentralized states. This duality persisted until the administration of Ernesto Zedillo (1994–2000), who proceeded to decentralize health service administration for the non-insured in all states, although retaining the separation between the IMSS-managed health infrastructure and the rest of the government services.

■ **2.1.8** *Conditional cash transfers*

Neoliberal in orientation, President Carlos Salinas de Gortari (1988–1994) downsized the state and eliminated COPLAMAR in the process. The IMSS-COPLAMAR programme became housed more directly under IMSS as part of a Solidarity Initiative, which coordinated cross-sectoral programmes and services with the aim of combating poverty through credit. Priority within the health system was given to achieving universal immunization coverage, in close collaboration across all public health institutions. The World Bank also supported basic health coverage extension programmes following WHO guidelines. President Ernesto Zedillo Ponce de León (1994–2000) introduced conditional cash transfers for education and health-based initiatives that required the compliance of at-risk populations to meet performance indicators, the so-called Health, Education and Nutrition Programme (PROGRESA). Families in extreme poverty were identified, registered and entitled to receive cash benefits conditional on attendance of health promotion sessions and maintaining their children in school.

■ **2.1.9** *Rise and demise of Seguro Popular*

The year 2000 saw the rise to power of the first opposition party president since the Revolution, Vicente Fox Quezada (2000–2006). Subsequent health policy focused on achieving universal financial protection to reduce catastrophic health expenditures, a policy aligned with the WHO's World Health Report 2000, and supporting the realization of the constitutional right to health protection. Article 77 of the General Health Law was amended to establish the System for Social Protection in Health (SPSS) which funded Seguro Popular – a new coverage programme for the uninsured. Initiated in 2003, SPSS comprises a financial model emulating tripartite social insurance funding: 1) the federal government finances a fixed "social fee" per person registered with Seguro Popular, financed mainly out of increasing oil revenues; 2) state governments contribute half of this amount as a *pari passu*; 3) those insured above the poverty level contribute an annual fee that varies according to income. The formation of Seguro Popular was aimed to reduce financial disparities among the uninsured across states as well between the uninsured and insured (Knaul & Frenk, 2005; González Pier et al., 2005).

SPSS increased total public health expenditure while reducing out-of-pocket expenditure, incentivized state government contributions, reduced inequity between the insured and uninsured and across states with differing levels of development, and increased expenditure on medicines and investment with respect to human resources. An explicit package of services was established, covering most primary care and general hospital interventions as well as selected high-cost or "catastrophic" interventions. Funding and provision were decoupled and placed under separate administrations, with the possibility of contracting from public or private providers outside state or federal government providers. This structure was intended to assure quality by requiring provider accreditation prior to funding and also through voluntary registration by beneficiaries, which would act as a stimulus for infrastructure maintenance and to ensure the satisfaction of beneficiaries and hence their continued membership in the system.

SPSS was implemented gradually during the administrations of Presidents Fox and his successor Felipe Calderón Hinojosa (2006–2012). During this time, the uninsured decreased from 49.6% of the total population in 2000 to 17.3% in 2015, while coverage of high-cost interventions expanded from six interventions in 2000 to 66 for December 2018, with the latest inclusions being oesophageal cancer and heart, liver and lung transplants (CNPSS, 2018b). The age limit for highly prevalent myocardial infarction (heart attack) was expanded from adults under 60 to under 65. Kidney transplant for adults and haemodialysis for terminal kidney disease remain uncovered. On the financial front, total public health expenditure increased by about 1% of GDP, rising from 5% in 2000 to 6.3% in 2014, while out-of-pocket expenditure decreased from 55% of total health expenditure to 43.2%.

During the Calderón administration, a strategy of insurance portability and quality standard convergence was undertaken with the aim of increasing the coordination across public provider institutions. Agreements were signed across institutions to exchange services within a limited set of specialized interventions to rationalize the utilization of infrastructure and reduce the need for investments. The economic downturn of 2009 was addressed through cost containment and the consolidated purchasing of drugs for most public institutions. In 2014 efforts were made to curb financial mismanagement by state health authorities through changes to the General Health Law, whereby the federation recentralized resource management and implemented measures to strengthen accountability at state level.

In spite of its advanced financial architecture, SPSS encountered limitations reaching its stated aims. Transparency and accountability were limited, particularly at state level, leading to uncertainty in resource allocation and to fraud in some cases (see section 7.1.1). As affiliation into the system reached its potential, state health authorities lost incentives to maintain quality which led to the persistence of problems such as insufficient resource allocation and low satisfaction (see section 6.7). Furthermore, SPSS only partially achieved its aim of shifting funding from the supply side, based on historical funding, to the demand side, based on performance-based payments (see section 6.4). While inequalities were reduced across states and between urban and rural areas, differences persisted (see section 7.2). Catastrophic health expenditures by households were reduced; however, a small but still significant portion of the population remained uninsured (see section 7.3). While the proportion of the uninsured fell to 14.6%, the remaining gap, as well as explicit service restrictions for those covered by Seguro Popular, reveals that the health system has failed to achieve universal health coverage. Finally, the high rates of rotation between the formal and informal labour markets led to complex financing arrangements that weakened demand-side funding (see section 7.7.1). Some of these shortcomings were addressed by the Peña Nieto administration, particularly the lack of accountability.

The shortcomings in the SPSS and particularly the explicit restriction of services covered and the gap in the uninsured were the basis of its demise in November 2019 and substitution by the Policy for Free Health Services and Medicines, to be operated by a new Institute for Health for Wellbeing (INSABI). The new policy is based on the right to health protection enshrined by the Constitution in 1983 and aims to provide the same range of services as IMSS, although through a separate infrastructure. The aim is for INSABI to integrate funding and provision while centralizing health services financing, taking them away from state health providers. Nonetheless, state governments' responsibilities as health authorities and health providers have not been modified. INSABI aims to establish fully funded, integrated public health networks, cancelling all private subcontracting. A population register will be established, not as an instrument of affiliation – a resource allocation mechanism that is to disappear – but rather as an accountability mechanism (see sections 2.3.1 and 2.6.1).

■ 2.2 **Organization**

The Mexican health system consists of three main subsystems operating in parallel, each responsible for funding, service provision and, to a large extent, regulation. Coverage for the poor and uninsured is organized by INSABI at the federal level on the basis of the General Health Law and with collaboration by state governments, to cover about 43.5% of the population. Social insurance institutions are governed at the federal level through their own laws, providing health care and broader social security benefits, such as pensions, to those formally employed, which amount to about 40.4% of the population. Finally, there is a private subsystem that is organized through market principles (Figure 2.1). The MoH regulates specific functions and with variable authority across the three subsystems. Government health services for the uninsured are mostly organized through agreements for funding and collaboration across the federal and state governments. An important exception is IMSS-Bienestar, a federal programme that funds IMSS to provide basic health care to the rural poor through a separate network of clinics and hospitals. In practice, the health system is a patchwork of diverse and often overlapping principles and legal charters.

The government services for the non-insured and social insurance institutions have assumed the responsibility to fund and to directly provide most health care services, purchasing inputs from the private sector and contracting-out services only when faced with significant shortages or when restrictions to investment have made it necessary. As of 2020, current policy in fact aims to substitute all private sector subcontracting with public provision (Secretaría de Salud, 2019). The private sector is constituted mostly of small firms, with a few large national corporations primarily in the hospital and pharmaceutical sectors and a large multinational pharmaceutical sector. The private sector is organized to varying degrees through national health provision, manufacturing, distribution and commercialization associations. Private health service providers are mostly funded through out-of-pocket expenditure and less so through private health insurance; the latter contracts mostly from the large hospitals in the private sector. The growth, investment and business logic of the private health care actors has depended mainly on the monopolistic tendencies and insufficient capacity of public payers and providers.

FIG. 2.1 Organization of the Mexican health system according to funding, provision and population coverage

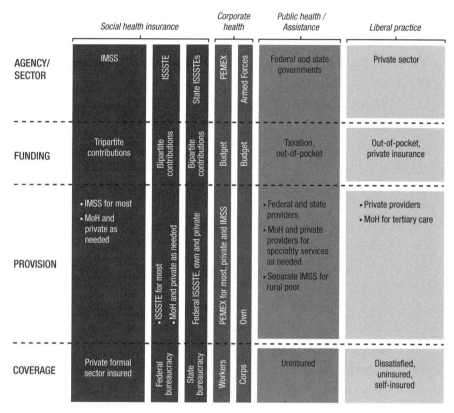

Note: Column width indicates approximate relative size of funding, provision and coverage

Source: Authors

2.2.1 *Federal level*

At the federal level, the Congress and Senate, MoH, the Federal Commission for the Protection Against Sanitary Risks (COFEPRIS) and the General Health Council are the key actors in the health care system. The General Health Law introduced the notion of a National Health System as a mechanism to enable the MoH's coordination of the diverse entities in the health system. This law established voluntary committees and commissions that bring together state authorities and social insurance institutions, and to some extent the private sector.

The MoH is organized into three undersecretaries and six national or federal commissions (Secretaría de Salud, 2018a):

- Undersecretary for Administration and Financing;
- Undersecretary for Health Sector Integration and Development;
- Undersecretary for Health Prevention and Promotion;
- National Commission Against Addictions;
- National Commission for National Institutes of Health and High Specialty Hospitals (CINSHAE);
- Federal Commission for the Protection Against Sanitary Risks (COFEPRIS);
- Institute for Health for Wellbeing (INSABI);
- National Commission for Bioethics;
- National Commission for Medical Arbitration.

In addition, the MoH is supported by other federal entities including the Coordinating Unit for Linkage and Social Participation, the Unit for Economic Analysis, the National Health Council, the Organs for Internal Control and the Legal Department. The MoH coordinates the General Health Council, a body that is legally dependent on the president, who appoints its head. The General Health Council includes 13 members from other branches of the federal government and from NGOs, all appointed by the president.

PAYERS

The federal government funds tertiary care and transfers funds to states for first and second level providers of care through three mechanisms: CINSHAE, the Undersecretary for Administration and Financing and INSABI. CINSHAE funds federal tertiary care hospitals mainly through historical budgets covering all line items and through performance incentives tied to research. The Undersecretary for Administration and Financing directly funds the historical budget to cater to the uninsured through national institutes and hospitals and state-level health systems organized in collaboration with state governments, covering mostly personnel and infrastructure.

Until its demise in 2019, CNPSS paid for about half of the personal health services of the uninsured population enrolled in Seguro Popular, mostly provided by federal institutes and hospitals and by state-level health provider networks. The funding covered two main benefits packages: essential services, as defined by the Universal Health Services Catalogue (CAUSES), and high-cost specialty services as defined by the Protection Fund for Catastrophic Health Expenditures (FPGC). CAUSES funding was transferred to the states according to a formula that allocates resources based on the number of people enrolled in Seguro Popular by the State Regimens for Social Protection in Health (REPSS), the bodies charged with allocating federal and state funds to the state-level provider network. FPGC covered a list of 66 high-specialty interventions and was paid directly by the federal government's CNPSS to accredited providers (see sections 3.2.2 and 3.3.1) (González Block et al., 2018c). Funding for the two packages was allocated mostly to state or federal providers, with a small part allocated to accredited private providers, mostly for highly specialized interventions.

From 2020, INSABI is expected to allocate funding formerly assigned by Seguro Popular and the National Commission for Social Protection in Health. It is not yet clear how state funding will be administered, as it is no longer a requirement for INSABI allocations. Furthermore, it is not clear how federal transfers to state governments following historical budgets will be managed, although it is expected that they will continue after an approval process by INSABI. The General Health Law now mandates INSABI to ensure the federal budget to be based on a historical basis, that is, to be allocated each year on the basis of the previous year, adjusted for inflation. This means that funding will no longer follow the people affiliated to a formal scheme such as Seguro Popular, even if this population may decrease as social insurance affiliation increases. INSABI will maintain an earmarked fund for catastrophic health expenditures, such as was the case for FPGC with Seguro Popular. INSABI has committed to maintain funding for the same diseases covered and to gradually expand coverage until there are no differences with respect to social insurance institutions. However, it is not clear if provider payment will be on a per-service basis as before, or if public providers will receive additional funds through their annual budgeting processes.

The MoH and social insurance institutions together with the National Science and Technology Council (CONACYT) also funded the Sectoral Fund for Research in Health and Social Security (FOSISS) until 2018. Together they allocated funds through yearly competitive calls for applications open to all registered public and private institutions, provided that IMSS and MoH researchers were the main beneficiaries.

PROVIDERS

CINSHAE is responsible for overseeing the funding and coordination of 13 National Institutes of Health, each specializing in different clinical areas, and six Federal Reference Hospitals. These institutes and hospitals are all located in Mexico City except for the National Institute of Public Health. CINSHAE also coordinates six regional High Specialty Hospitals positioned in key cities across the country. These federal facilities provide mostly tertiary clinical care and constitute the country's main basic and clinical research infrastructure. Moreover, these federal facilities mostly provide clinical care for the uninsured, although the insured can also access these facilities on a fee-for-service (FFS) basis. CINSHAE also funds and coordinates health research at the federal level in collaboration with CONACYT. The federal government also oversees a network of state or federally owned national reference laboratories.

2.2.2 *State level*

Each of the 32 states is responsible for health regulation and health service provision according to the General Health Law, mostly through state-owned general hospitals and primary care units. State and federal authorities share responsibilities for sanitary regulation and personal health services for Mexicans who are not covered by any of the employment-based social insurance schemes run by corporatist health institutions. State health laws were decreed in the 1980s modelled on the federal General Health Law as a means of aligning collaboration across the two orders of government. The federal government and states signed yearly collaboration agreements to receive federal funding for Seguro Popular and it is expected agreements will also be signed from 2020 to receive INSABI funding. However, it is not yet clear how state revenue coming from transfers from the federal government – which constitute the majority of their health funds – will be managed and the role INSABI will have in such a process.

Ministries of health at the state level are led by a state government-appointed minister and tend to mirror the federal MoH. Since 1995, all states proceeded to decentralize health service provision through state-delegated autonomous entities governed by boards with official participation by both levels of government (see section 2.1.7). Beginning in 2014, State Regimens for Social Protection in Health (REPSS) were transformed into state-delegated autonomous bodies tasked with managing the financial resources of SPSS, pooling resources assigned by the CNPSS and by state governments as well as family contributions. While this arrangement introduced the separation of functions between funding and provision at the state level, over half of federal funding was still allocated directly by the federal government to state treasuries to pay for human resources and other obligations (González Block, 2017). REPSS disappeared in 2020 and INSABI proceeded to directly allocate state funds or to direct administration by state ministries of health through coordination agreements.

■ **2.2.3** *Corporatist arrangements*

Social insurance institutions are governed by Article 123 of the Constitution. Section A of the Article establishes the rights of private sector employees, legislated through the Social Insurance Law governing the IMSS. Fraction B establishes the rights of government employees and is legislated through the ISSSTE. The labour rights of state and municipal government employees are protected by state constitutions, but ISSSTE or IMSS can provide health and social services under agreement for those states that have not established their own social insurance institutes for the purpose. ISSSTE covers all branches of the federal government as well as autonomous and parastatal organs and includes the government employees of Mexico City. In addition to IMSS and ISSSTE, the federal Secretariats of National Defence and the Navy as well as the Mexican Petroleum Company (PEMEX) provide health services to their forces or employees.

Both IMSS and ISSSTE are decentralized, autonomous entities of the federal government and are regulated through their own laws and governing assemblies, while vertically integrating fund collection, pooling, purchasing and provision.

TRADE UNIONS IN THE HEALTH SECTOR

Professional and ancillary employees of government health institutions are affiliated with large, institution-specific trade unions established and controlled by the federal government since their inception in 1943. IMSS has the largest and most privileged workforce, with 333 000 active and 246 000 retired workers. Over half a million trade union affiliates are politically active, as pensions are critical for both active workers and retirees. Pensions are adjusted based on employee salary negotiations and not on inflation. Furthermore, the pension fund for workers contracted prior to 1995 and including 50% of the total – the Retirement and Pensions Scheme (*Régimen de Jubilaciones y Pensiones*; RJP) – enables pensioners to retire 12 years younger and with pensions eight times higher than those of the workers they protect. Furthermore, retirees receive 29% higher income than workers. Critically, the RJP is bankrupt, with only 4.6% of the funding required to meet its obligations and leading it to absorb 19% of operational income, a figure that is expected to reach 63% by 2034 (González Block 2018). The IMSS trade union is highly combative of initiatives suggesting sectoral integration or even coordination in the context of increasing financial pressures within the RJP. The government, for its part, is reluctant to address these issues as the levelling of privileges across health sector trade unions is not viable. Policies, thus, are limited to expanding the coverage of private sector workers by IMSS while reducing investments and proposing weak sector coordination strategies with other health institutions (see section 6.6.5).

BENEFITS AND SERVICE PROVISION

Social insurance institutions provide a full range of promotional, preventive, curative and rehabilitation services, with few exclusions and no defined benefit packages. Institutions cover specific risks through separate funds. In the case of IMSS these are Occupational Risk Insurance (SRT); Sickness and Maternity Insurance (SEM); Incapacity and Life Insurance (SIV);

Retirement, Cessation in Old Age and Old Age Insurance (SRCV); and Infant Care Insurance and Social Benefits (SGPS). ISSSTE and state institutes offer a similar range of benefits according to their own laws. IMSS, however, entitles beneficiaries to different benefit packages or to different contribution rules, distinguishing up to 15 different categories (Table 2.1).

In most cases, social insurance institutions own their health infrastructure and hire salaried employees, who are mostly unionized through institutional trade unions. Basic health services are organized in tiered networks of primary care and general hospitals organized at state levels. Tertiary care services are organized through decentralized, semi-autonomous hospitals governed by boards constituted by government, employer and employee representatives in the case of IMSS, and by government representatives in the case of MoH. ISSSTE tertiary care hospitals are managed centrally. In the state of Baja California, IMSS, ISSSTE and the MoH co-own a specialty hospital, which is a unique circumstance resulting from the state's isolation.

IMSS also has a limited number of funding agreements with the banking industry and selected industrial, mining and agricultural companies and organizations (*reversión de cuotas*), enabling them to directly provide health services for their employees through their own or contracted services, for which IMSS reimburses part of the employer and employee insurance contributions. These agreements are a historical remnant and new agreements are conceded by IMSS only to firms whose geographical isolation prevents IMSS from establishing its own services (see section 3.2.2).

FINANCING AND COST CONTAINMENT

Social insurance institutions are funded through contributions from the government, employers and employees, with the government also contributing in its capacity as employer in the cases of ISSSTE and state social insurance institutions. Government contributions consist of two parts: 1) a contribution based on employee earnings, and 2) a social fee assessed as a fixed amount per employee. Employee contributions vary by scheme and are proportional to earnings up to a ceiling, while in the case of IMSS, low-earning employees are exempted from contributions.

TABLE 2.1 IMSS insurance according to regimen, contribution modality and benefit scheme, 2014

CATEGORY AND REGIMEN	POPULATION INSURED	%	SRT	SEM	SIV	SRCV	SGPS
Obligatory regimen							
Permanent and temporary workers in cities	17 573 914	67.9	X	X	X	X	X
Direct service provision by employers (banking industry and selected industrial, mining and agricultural companies)	319 001	1.2	X	X	X	X	X
Permanent and temporary workers in rural areas	41 021	0.2	X	X	X	X	X
Temporary sugar cane workers	100 815	0.4	X	X	X	X	X
Permanent sugar cane workers	98 236	0.4	X	X	X	X	
Subtotal	**18 132 987**	**70.1**					
Voluntary regime							
Facultative insurance (students and others)	6 818 123	26.3		X			
Family health insurance (individuals outside the obligatory and facultative regimes)	315 592	1.2		X			
Voluntary continuation in the obligatory regime (for employees that end their employment)	133 142	0.5			X	X	
Independent workers (self-employed)	31 052	0.1		X	X	X	
Domestic workers	3359	0.0	X	X	X	X	
Employees employed by other individuals (not firms)	6443	0.0	X	X	X	X	
State, municipal and decentralized organism employees[a]	151 050	0.6		X			
Federal, state and municipal employees[a]	254 657	1.0	X	X			
Federal, state and municipal employees[a]	14 503	0.1	X	X	X	X	
Voluntary incorporation of rural workers to the obligatory regime	22 573	0.1		X	X	X	
Subtotal	**7 750 494**	**29.9**					
TOTAL	**25 883 481**	**100**					

SRT, Occupational risk insurance; SEM, Sickness and maternity insurance; SIV, Incapacity and life insurance; SRCV, Retirement, cessation (loss of employment) in old age; SGPS, Infant care insurance and social benefits

[a]Schemes differ only in the benefits provided according to agreements with public institutions. The orange shading indicates when the insurance includes economic benefits, and not only medical care

Sources: Modified from IMSS (2017), p. 48; IMSS (2014), Annex A

Social insurance institutions have addressed cost containment mostly through reducing consumable and pharmaceutical costs. IMSS was charged by President Calderón with organizing drug purchasing for all public institutions willing to pool their resources. To this end, IMSS consolidates annual purchases under a single national process and establishes a reverse-bidding procedure to reduce provider prices. Patent medicines are purchased through sector-wide negotiations with pharmaceutical companies undertaken by the Coordinating Commission for Negotiating the Price of Medicines and other Health Inputs (CCPNMIS), based on international reference prices. Other cost-containment and revenue-increasing measures have been introduced through administrative simplification and the financial management of reserves. These measures have attained a modicum of success, with the nominal budgetary allocation for medicine reducing by about 6% per annum since 2012. However, actual cost reductions have been more modest – in the order of 1%, which is partly due to the fact that some distributors fail to deliver on the agreed prices (Health Research Institute, 2017).

GOVERNANCE

IMSS is governed through an assembly and a technical council, both charged with executive functions. The assembly approves an annual general plan as proposed by the technical council, while this latter body oversees its execution on a day-to-day basis. The assembly is made up of 30 members designated in equal parts by three constituencies: the federal government, official trade unions and official employer organizations. Assembly members are elected from within the ranks of four trade unions and two employer organizations for renewable 6-year terms. Similarly, the assembly nominates 12 members to the technical council, four from each constituency. Federal government members from the finance, labour and health ministries participate ex officio, with the additional participation of a president-appointed IMSS director, who chairs the council.

The federal government selects the organizations participating in the IMSS assembly and technical council according to their size, although they have remained mostly unchanged since the 1940s. The employer representatives are designated by the Confederation of Chambers of Industry of Mexico (CONCAMIN) – with three members – and the Confederation of National

Chambers of Commerce and Tourism (CONCANACO-SERVYTUR) – with one member. Both organizations were originally chartered by federal law to be the exclusive representatives with the federal government of any legally-constituted chamber. However, obligatory membership was discontinued in early 2000 in a relaxation of vertical corporatism. Employee confederations include the most powerful, yet waning, trade unions traditionally allied to the government and the ruling party. Independent trade unions are thus not represented in spite of their growing size. Both employer and employee confederations directly represent a small minority of IMSS insured, with only 6.9% belonging to a trade union in 2017 and 3.1% to the unions represented in the confederations that participate in the governing board (González Block, 2018).

ISSSTE is governed through a board of directors constituted by 19 members, including the president-appointed director and chair. The Ministry of Treasury and Public Credit appoints three members, while the ministries of Health, Social Development, Labour, Environment and Natural Resources, Comptroller General and IMSS appoint their minister or director. Labour organizations appoint the nine remaining representatives.

2.2.4 *Private sector*

Mexico's private health subsystem is large and growing, mainly as a response to the limitations of the public sector within the context of an increasingly competitive economy and an ageing population. Government health providers should meet most of the population's health needs according to their charters. However, underfunding and inefficiency have led to government health service shortages, providing the private sector with an opportunity for their fulfilment. Private providers are also the main source of care for the uninsured. Up to 45% of total outpatient consultations and 19.5% of hospital care is supplied by private providers. Among the patients covered by social insurance institutions, up to 32% of outpatient care and 14.1% of hospital care is provided by private providers. In the case of the non-insured, up to 33% of total outpatient consultations and 14.8% of hospital care is supplied by private providers. Public health care services are preferred for the more costly care while the private sector is often the first choice of care for minor conditions as well as for continued care among the wealthy, particularly those covered by private health insurance (González Block et al., 2018b).

Private providers and private insurance are segmented according to Mexico's socioeconomic strata. Some 83% of Mexican households situated in socioeconomic strata E (extremely poor) to C (below the poverty line) have – to varying degrees – geographical access to 52 200 general physicians, mostly in solo practice, practising in small towns to large urban areas. A majority of these physicians are pharmacy chain employees and provide their services at low cost in consulting rooms adjacent to the pharmacies. The population represented in these strata also has geographically varying access to 2829 hospitals nationally, of which 2400 are up to 14 beds in size and the rest between 15 and 49 beds. Private providers supply between 18–33% of ambulatory care and 10–27% of hospital care across strata E to C, paying mostly out-of-pocket (González Block et al., 2018b).

The more advantaged households (in socioeconomic strata C+ to A, making up 17% of households) are catered to by 15 500 independent specialist physicians mostly through self-referral. Specialists are increasingly located in consultation clinics adjacent to the country's 94 largest private hospitals, which serve as their primary source of referrals for high-technology analyses and admissions. Up to 27% of the population in strata C+ to A are privately insured, mostly through policies reimbursing hospital expenses. Private health insurance covers mostly private hospital care, although privately insured patients accessing highly specialized MoH institutes are also reimbursed. Private insurance is estimated to save IMSS and ISSSTE up to 7.6% of their total hospital costs by funding private care for those patients who are also privately insured (González Block et al., 2018b).

■ 2.3 Decentralization and centralization

The Mexican health system is governed and managed through a mix of decentralized and centralized policies and systems. The federal government is responsible for the general health of the population, understood chiefly as the prevention of risks that cross states such as those related to industrialized products and epidemics. Governance of health services for the non-insured also falls under General Health as an area of shared responsibility between federal and state governments. On the other hand, health services for the insured under social insurance institutions are excluded from General Health and are thus outside the remit of the Ministry of Health (see sections 2.1.4 and 2.2.3).

■ 2.3.1 *Health services for the non-insured*

The federal government and state governments have had signed collaboration agreements to coordinate their health responsibilities and funding since the 1930s. The federal government has assumed greater responsibility to fund and provide personal health services for the uninsured and the poor through SPSS and Seguro Popular, more so now with INSABI. While SPSS started as a cash-transfer programme to state governments, corruption and state government inefficiency led to recentralized financial control in 2014 by mandating states to manage at least 50% of funding through Federal Treasury (Tesofe) accounts. Furthermore, REPSS were mandated to be established as decentralized state government bodies and at arm's length from state health providers – enabling them to have a more direct relationship with the federal CNPSS and thus providing federal authorities with greater control over state financial management (González Block et al., 2018c). While Tesofe accounts will be maintained by INSABI, it is expected that funding through this channel will be reduced as INSABI pays a greater share of resources directly to providers.

While state governments increased their absolute financial contributions to health care for the uninsured as part of the conditionality imposed by SPSS, funding remains mostly federal, and the relative share of state governments' total public spending on the uninsured actually decreased from 15.2% in 2000 to 13.1% in 2014 (González Block et al., 2018c). It is uncertain how state funding will evolve under INSABI, but given the ending of conditional cash transfers, it may be reduced.

Decentralization of services for the non-insured has been limited since its inception in the 1980s, retaining a high level of federal funding regardless of the states' income levels. This is particularly the case given the high level of human resource contracting by the federal government, and their consequent unionization at the federal level. State ministries of health have thus not evolved their policy-making and administrative capacities, while the federation has further centralized financial control. Under INSABI, the architecture of health services for the non-insured will revert in essence to the situation existing prior to 1983.

The National Health Council was established in 1988 to coordinate policy-making across decentralized state ministries of health. However, the Council was reformed in 2013 to also include representatives from social insurance institutions in an effort to strengthen sector-wide coordination. State Health Councils have a similar composition and support health sector development at this level. The private sector is not represented in either body, reflecting the dependency private actors have with respect to public institutions.

■ **2.3.2** *Centralized governance of social insurance*

The Constitution gives powers to the federal government to fund and manage social insurance institutions through highly centralized, corporatist arrangements (see section 2.2.3). These functions are undertaken by IMSS and ISSSTE as entities with delegated powers, but also through health institutions within the military and the navy as well as within PEMEX. As mentioned above, IMSS was established through the Social Insurance Law of 1943 as a delegated corporatist organization funded and governed through tripartite arrangements. Governance is through an assembly and a technical council, each integrated by equal numbers of federal government, employers and employee representatives. The nominating organizations, which have remained unchanged since the 1940s and 1950s, were designated by the federal government from the most numerous as well as officially recognized organizations. The director of IMSS is appointed by the president and chairs both the assembly and the technical council. The agenda is mostly set by the federal government, which identifies the social groups that need to be incorporated into IMSS as well as the financial policies to be pursued.

2.4 **Intersectorality**

The Mexican government has developed intersectoral health strategies and programmes with the ministries of Health, Social Development and Government being chiefly responsible for coordination and implementation.

The most important areas for intersectoral collaboration have been population policy, poverty and the epidemics of diabetes, overweight and obesity. Among the oldest intersectoral programmes is family planning, established in the 1970s by the National Council on Population (CONAPO) which led communication and health campaigns to reduce fertility rates. CONAPO currently prioritizes the prevention of teen pregnancy as well as the sexual abuse of minors in close coordination with the MoH and the Ministry of Government.

The Ministry of Welfare runs specific programmes to improve maternal and child health and nutrition in communities under extreme poverty. The most salient programme is Bienestar (previously known as the Health, Education and Nutrition Programme, PROGRESA, then as *Oportunidades* and up until January 2019 as *Prospera*), first implemented in 1997 as a conditional cash-transfer programme to provide monetary incentives to families to comply with health promotion initiatives and keep their children at school and delivers food assistance to designated families. The programme's impact on health and nutrition have been positively evaluated (INSP/CIESAS, 2008).

The MoH coordinates the Programme for Healthy Environments and Communities, which empowers local intersectoral committees to improve well-being by focusing on social determinants of health and through the training of health promotors. The private sector has attempted to develop its own brand of intersectoral programming and in 2009 established the Council for Self-Regulation and Advertisement Ethics (CONAR), which promoted the Self-Regulation of Food and Non-Alcoholic Drink Advertisement Directed to Child Audiences (PABI). Over 30 of Mexico's largest food processing companies committed to PABI, yet according to the National Institute of Public Health, PABI does not comply with WHO standards as it allows for highly attractive advertisement campaigns regardless of nutritional criteria and fails to specify the media channels to be regulated (INSP, 2013).

To curb diabetes, obesity and overweight, in 2014 the Ministry of the Treasury implemented a special tax on sugary drinks and foods with high caloric content. The tax has been positively evaluated in its impact on sugary drink consumption (Colchero et al., 2015; 2017) (see section 5.1.4). From 2014 and up until its demise in 2019, the MoH led a National Strategy on Diabetes, Obesity and Overweight and established a council with public–private representation for the purpose. The strategy focuses on public health campaigns promoting nutritional habits, exercise and medical check-ups. Another important initiative was the Ministry of Education's prohibition starting in 2014 of the sale of high-sugar foods and drinks in primary schools. The strategy also aimed at improving the quality of care and prevention within MoH facilities, mostly through developing information systems in collaboration with the private Carlos Slim Foundation (FCS).

Finally, the MoH implements other programmes with a broad inter-sectoral focus, such as against addictions, towards the prevention of traffic accidents and to promote the health of migrant workers who frequently travel to and from the United States.

■ 2.5 **Health information systems**

Mexico's health information system is regulated by the National Institute of Statistics and Geography (INEGI) through specialized technical committees tasked with integrating health information. Recent developments include the 2004 MoH decree, the Official Mexican Standard for Health Information, followed in 2009 by the Specialized Technical Committee for Sectoral Health Information, established under the presidency of the MoH's General Directorate for Health Information (DGIS), with the participation of all public institutions and representatives of the private sector. DGIS is affiliated with the Collaborating Centres for the WHO Family of International Classifications and is the national authority responsible for health sector classifications. Among other functions, DGIS established the national standards for the system of electronic clinical records.

Health information at the national level is available through three main sources: 1) the annual federal executive government report; 2) the annual report on the Health of Mexicans; and 3) the National Health and Nutrition Survey (ENSANUT) reports, produced every 5 years. The annual executive government report describes the actions and strategies carried out during the year, in relation to the Health Sector Programme published at the beginning of each federal administration. The reports on the Health of Mexicans (published only in 2015 and 2016) offer a general assessment of the health system on the basis of administrative data covering financing, resources, provision of services and quality. All evaluation reports carried out by the National Council for the Evaluation of Social Development Policy (CONEVAL) or the MoH are published online by the General Directorate for Performance Evaluation (DGED). The ENSANUT – last published in 2019 – generate national- and state-level reports that summarize the main indicators of public health as well as on the performance of the health system. The National Epidemiological Surveillance System (SINAVE) has published statistical yearbooks since 1984 as well as weekly epidemiological bulletins that report on new cases of 142 diseases. Hospital diagnosis and discharge statistics are another national source of morbidity data and have been compiled by the Automated Hospital Discharge Subsystem (SAEH).

The National Health Information System (SINAIS) collects, monitors and disseminates health information through five subsystems:

- population and coverage
- human, physical, material and financial resources
- health services
- health situation
- performance evaluation.

SINAIS integrates all public and private provider units under a single catalogue with a Unique Health Establishment Code (CLUES) specifying their level of care and material resources available. The System for Health Care Equipment, Human Resources and Infrastructure (SINERHIAS) complements CLUES by providing a comprehensive facility catalogue. SINAVE is operated on the Unique Epidemiological Surveillance Information System (SUIVE) platform. SUIVE collates weekly epidemiological reports provided by all medical care units. The MoH is also the primary authority for the issuance of birth certificates and is the source of information on live births. Health expenditure information is collected through national surveys and fed into the National Health Accounts Information System (SICUENTAS).

In 2012, the MoH updated the Official Mexican Standard for Health Information leading to the establishment of the National Basic Health Information System (SINBA) aimed at improving the exchange and analysis of health information at the national level. SINBA integrates SINAIS and SUIVE into a single system with protocols designed to improve reporting, integration, analysis and evaluation by public and private institutions. SINBA is being rolled out and intends to provide a unique personal identifier to all residents through which to track coverage and care as well as to facilitate the transfer of medical records and other nominal information across institutions. It is anticipated that the quality of information should also be improved through more timely and more consistent reporting.

The MoH monitors public health through three administrative units: 1) the General Directorate for Health Information (DGIS) coordinates the statistical information system; 2) the General Directorate of Epidemiology is responsible for SINAVE; and 3) the General Directorate for Performance Evaluation (DGED) is the coordinating and normative body for the evaluation of the subsystems that make up the National Health System. Furthermore, external bodies contribute to the generation and official validation of health information, chief among them INEGI and CONAPO. INEGI presides over Mexico's Statistical and Geographic Information System, including all information related to resources, population and the economy. In addition to its activities with respect to fertility, CONAPO is responsible for demographic analysis, evaluation and systematization through the collaboration of 17 federal public administration agencies chaired by the minister of the interior.

■ 2.6 **Regulation and planning**

■ **2.6.1** *Principal policy orientations*

The Constitution enshrines the right to health protection in Article 4, differentiating health service access and privileges according to Article 123 which enshrines social security rights exclusively for workers in the public and private labour markets. Article 73 of the Constitution empowers Congress to enact social insurance legislation as its exclusive responsibility, bypassing state governments. However, Article 4 allocates joint responsibility for the right to health protection to state and federal governments. The Constitution also recognizes the human rights enshrined in ratified international treaties, including the "right of everyone to the enjoyment of the highest attainable standard of physical and mental health" enshrined by the International Covenant on Economic, Social and Cultural Rights (see Table 2.2).

TABLE 2.2 Responsibilities for specific health system functions according to levels of care in the Mexican health system

SECTOR	COVERAGE DECISIONS	LICENSING/ACCREDITATION
Ambulatory and inpatient care	Right to health protection chartered in the Constitution through federal and corporatist principles. Coverage entitlements with respect to health benefits are set implicitly, with exclusions defined only in social insurance laws and regulations. Explicit coverage entitlements were specified by the General Health Law for the uninsured according to CAUSES and FPGC. INSABI will determine new lists through gradual expansion. Federal and state hospitals provide services outside lists reimbursed through means-tested out-of-pocket payments. It is uncertain how such charges will evolve under INSABI. Private insurers set own coverage schemes.	Health professionals licensed by the Ministry of Education upon graduation. Medical specialties accredited by specialty councils. Facility accreditation by MoH-COFEPRIS for general operational permits and voluntary quality accreditation by the GHC. MoH-DGCES accredited quality standards within MoH to enable funding by CNPSS. Under INSABI, plans are underway to transfer accreditation to the General Health Council.
Pharmaceutical (ambulatory)	From 2019, the General Health Council established a National Compendium of Health Inputs homogenizing lists across institutions. However, each social insurance institution and INSABI will purchase according to needs and possibilities based on budgets and own cost–effectiveness studies. Physicians determine drugs to be reimbursed by private insurers.	COFEPRIS licenses pharmaceutical manufacturing, distribution and dispensation. NHC approves pharmaceuticals for public use based on cost–effectiveness.
Public health services	National priorities and programmes set by MoH. State health authorities and local-level health jurisdictions supervise programmes.	None

CONTRACTUAL RELATIONSHIP BETWEEN SOCIAL INSURANCE INSTITUTIONS AND STATE AUTHORITIES, AND PROVIDERS	QUALITY ASSURANCE	FINANCING DECISIONS
Trade unions for each social insurance institution negotiate single collective contracts for health and non-health personnel. MoH and state employee trade unions govern health worker collective contracts nationally or at state levels.	General Health Law provides guidelines. MoH-CENETEC and DGCES coordinate clinical practice guidelines and norms. Obligatory implementation by federal and state agencies and voluntary implementation by social insurance institutions and private providers. MoH-DGCES regulates Special Health Insurance Institutions (ISES).	General Health Law determines funding for federal and state providers serving the uninsured. Certificates of need required to develop federal and state facilities. Each Social Insurance Law determines contributions for services for the insured and makes independent investment decisions.
Each institution purchases directly through distributors, increasingly after collective negotiations. Voluntary recommended pricing for the private sector regulated by Ministry of Commerce.	Pharmacovigilance coordinated by COFEPRIS.	Each institution or state health authority purchases directly. Increasingly, consolidated purchasing by public institutions through IMSS as sole negotiator and purchaser. Patent medicine prices established through the Coordinating Commission for Negotiating the Price of Medicines and other Health Inputs.
None	MoH establishes programme-monitoring indicators. Quality-monitoring programme *Caminando a la Excelencia* benchmarks performance.	INSABI and state governments allocate funding to priority public health programmes operated by state ministries of health and local health jurisdictions. Social insurance institutions fund own programmes and collaborate for national health campaigns with MoH.

Source: Based on General Health Law

Title 6 of the Constitution is devoted to Labour and Social Welfare (*Trabajo y Previsión Social*, which could be also translated as "Labour and Social Assurance"). Article 123, Section A is devoted to private sector workers and includes four components addressing health as part of labour rights. Fraction V covers pregnant working women and child labour; Fraction XIV establishes obligatory and inviolable workers' compensation for occupational risks; and Fraction XXIX addresses social insurance:

> The Social Insurance Law (Ley del Seguro Social) is of public interest, and will include insurance for incapacity, old age, life, involuntary cessation from work, sickness and accidents, child care services and any other geared to the protection and well-being of workers, peasants, non-salaried personnel and other social sectors and their families.[*]

Fraction XXIX includes general and not only occupational health and entitles groups – not individuals – beyond the strict labour parameters when specifying "other social sectors and their families".

Article 73 of the Constitution determines the legislative faculties of Congress and Fraction XVI enables this legislative body to dictate laws regarding General Health (*Salubridad General*), as distinct from local health, which is the remit of each sovereign state. Fraction XVI establishes the responsibility of the General Health Council, an executive body directly under the orders of the president "without the intervention of any State Ministry, and its general dispositions will be obligatory in all the country". However, Fraction XVI also assigns the responsibility of responding to epidemics of grave magnitude or to invasion by exotic diseases to the MoH. This recognizes that, in practice, the General Health Council has become subordinate to the MoH, although in a severe crisis, such as the H1N1 epidemic of 2009, the president called upon this body to coordinate the response across government.

The General Health Law acknowledges the diverging rights accrued through social security protections, differentiating accordingly the scope of the regulatory powers of the MoH in regard to social assistance and the

---

[*] It is important to clarify that in Spanish "*Seguro*" is translated as "insurance" and not as "security", which is translated as "*seguridad*". The semantic difference is important because it pertains to the distinction between corporatist social insurance in the German tradition against social security in the British or American traditions.

private sector, on the one hand, and for social insurance institutions, on the other. The General Health Law defines in Title 1 "General Dispositions", Article 2, the right to health protection as including, among other aspects, the enjoyment of health and social assistance services for the timely and efficacious satisfaction of the needs of the population. Article 3 defines general health as including the organization, control and surveillance of health services provision and of public, private and social sector health establishments, with the exclusion of social insurance agencies. In their case, the MoH can only coordinate and evaluate actions related to public policies and cannot dictate measures upon them nor enforce general health norms and regulations.

Mexico's health system has been oriented since 1983 by the constitutional decree of health protection as a right and since 2000 by a broad policy objective of achieving universal health coverage in line with the constitutional right to health protection. Policy has been influenced by the WHO's World Health Report 2000 and particularly by structuring policy around the health system objectives of improving health and equity, being responsive to the legitimate expectations of the population, and fairness of financial contributions (Frenk, 2010). The Peña Nieto 2012–2018 administration pursued six policy objectives: 1) increase disease protection, promotion and prevention; 2) ensure effective access to quality health services; 3) reduce lifestyle-related health risks; 4) close health gaps across social groups and regions of the country; 5) ensure the generation and effective use of health resources; and 6) move forward in establishing a universal national health system under the stewardship of the MoH (Secretaría de Salud, 2013e).

The health system observed a broad policy consensus between 1983 and 2018, with important exceptions. The consensus was challenged between 2000 and 2006 by then Chief of Government of Mexico City Andrés Manuel López Obrador and his Secretary for Health Asa Cristina Laurell, who proposed a vision of a fully tax-funded, free at the point-of-care health system integrating financing and provision. At the national level, this vision would lead to the end of Seguro Popular as a system with separation of funding and provision functions, and its replacement by an implicit package of funded services. Since López Obrador became president in December 2018, this vision has been affirmed, and Seguro Popular has been replaced with a policy of free medicines and services through INSABI (see sections 2.1.9 and 6.1).

■ **2.6.2** *Regulation and planning at the federal level*

The General Health Law assigns responsibilities across the MoH, the General Health Council and COFEPRIS at the federal level, and to the states. The MoH has exclusive responsibilities for the formulation of official general health regulations and to verify their compliance, as well as the exclusive responsibility to organize, operate and supervise the following aspects of general health (Ley General de Salud, 1983, Chapter II):

- organization, control and surveillance of all health providers except those belonging to social insurance institutions;
- coordination, evaluation and follow-up of health services provided by social insurance institutions;
- the national programme for HIV/AIDS and sexually transmitted diseases;
- the prevention of the consumption of narcotics and psychoactive drugs and the programme against addictions;
- sanitary regulation of pharmaceuticals and devices, including their production, use and final disposition, and the facilities where they are produced and their advertisement;
- sanitary regulation of organs, body tissues and cells; and
- international health.

The MoH also has the following responsibilities:

- organize and operate health services under its charge;
- support states as needed to carry out their responsibilities for general health and to exercise extraordinary actions as needed;
- promote coordination of all actors and subsystems as part of a National Health System;
- regulate, develop, coordinate, evaluate and supervise social protection (coverage) in health;
- evaluate the country's general health; and
- coordination and surveillance of General Health regulations according to the General Health Law.

The MoH is responsible for ensuring the right to health protection as defined by the Constitution, and the General Health Law (Title 2, Chapter II, Article 5). According to the General Health Law, the MoH coordinates all subsystems as part of a National Health System. This includes the formulation and implementation of national health policy according to existing laws as well as the coordination of health programmes across branches and entities of public administration at the federal level. Coordination with the states is achieved through agreements to collaborate according to the competencies of each order of government, leading to the establishment of state health systems.

The MoH thus coordinates and regulates federal health services, the state health authorities and the private and social sectors involved in the delivery of health services and in the production of health inputs. While the MoH cannot enforce regulations upon social insurance institutions, these latter may voluntarily comply with national standards and participate in coordination committees to collaborate in the resourcing and development of health information platforms, clinical practice guidelines, and health research funding initiatives, among others.

The General Health Council is charged with the following functions, to:

- dictate measures against alcohol addiction and the sale and production of toxic substances, as well as against environmental pollution;
- manage lists of pharmaceutical processing establishments and of priority diseases as well as sources of ionizing radiation;
- advise on health research and human resource training programmes and projects, including new areas for development;
- prepare the Basic List of Health Sector Inputs (approvals based on cost–effectiveness, once the MoH has approved them for safety and efficacy);
- participate in the consolidation and functioning of the NHS and prepare suggestions and opinions to the federal executive on its efficiency and on the performance of the Health Sector Programme;
- propose to the health authorities the provision of recognitions and incentives for institutions and persons that distinguish themselves for their merits in favour of health;

- analyse legal dispositions in health matters and formulate reform proposals or additions to the same; and
- support the development of the NHS through interinstitutional committees of its own, most importantly the committee for generic medicines, devices and diagnostic auxiliaries.

COFEPRIS is a deconcentrated MoH body charged with sanitary regulation under the scope and limitations outlined by the General Health Law. It has direct control over all public and private health establishments with the important exception of those operated by social insurance institutions (Ley General de Salud, 1983, *Artículo 17 bis*). COFEPRIS is also tasked with undertaking health risk assessments and for the development of national policy against health risks. Further, it is responsible for enforcing these policies in health establishments (excluding social insurance establishments) and for regulating medicines and other inputs, organs and tissues, food and drinks, cosmetic products, cleaning products, tobacco, pesticides, toxic substances, biotechnological products, food supplements, and environmental control, occupational health and basic sanitation. COFEPRIS is also charged with formulating and enforcing sanitary regulation of goods, infrastructure and services, with the exception of social insurance institution health establishments and the procurement and processing of organs, tissues and cells, which are the province of specialized agencies.

2.6.3 *Regulation at the state level*

The General Health Law assigns the following responsibilities to state governments:

- medical care provision, particularly for the most vulnerable groups;
- financial protection against the costs of health care among the uninsured;
- maternal and child health and nutrition, visual and auditory health, family planning and mental health;
- organization, coordination and surveillance of the exercise of activities by health professionals and by technical and auxiliary personnel;

- promotion of human resource training through state-level policies and provisions;
- health research coordination and the control of research in humans, including the human genome;
- health information with respect to health conditions, resources and services;
- health education for the population;
- prevention, orientation, control and surveillance for nutrition, respiratory diseases, cardiovascular diseases and diseases attributable to tobacco;
- prevention and control of the harmful effects of environmental factors upon human health;
- occupational health and basic sanitation;
- prevention and control of transmissible and non-transmissible diseases and of accidents;
- rehabilitation and prevention of disability;
- social assistance;
- programmes against alcohol and tobacco;
- sanitary regulation of human corpses;
- integrated pain care (prevention, treatment and control).

The General Health Law ascribes joint responsibility to the federal and state governments for the prevention of narcotics, care of people suffering addictions and the prosecution of related crime. Both orders of government can strike agreements to coordinate their competencies with respect to the delivery of general health services. These may involve the organization, control and surveillance of health providers except those belonging to social insurance institutions; coordination, evaluation and follow-up of social insurance institutions; the prevention of narcotic and psychotropic substance use; and performance of all functions under the responsibility of COFEPRIS (Ley General de Salud, 1983, Article 17). Additionally, both orders of government determine funding agreements for social protection in health.

Agreements across orders of government specify the contribution of financial resources and obligation to allocate resources to specified activities. Agreements can lead to the establishment of decentralized organs with an advisory board and the participation of beneficiaries and health workers. The heads of such units are designated by the federal minister of health following the states' executive recommendation. The most important decentralized organs involve the state health services, charged with integrating federal and state resources for health provision and sanitary risk protection, and, until the demise of Seguro Popular, REPSS for the funding of health services.

2.6.4 *Regulation at the social insurance level*

Social insurance institutions integrate health service provision and financing and are also self-regulated according to the General Health Law. They are, therefore, fully responsible for the organization, control and health risk surveillance of health facilities and procedures. As previously noted in section 2.2.1, institutions respond voluntarily to MoH requests for the establishment of joint committees such as health information and drug approvals within the scope of the NHS. Health service quality regulation and control is undertaken through their own standards and procedures. While beneficiaries may lodge complaints with the National Commission for Medical Arbitration, its decisions are not binding for the parties involved. The ordinary courts are responsible for the resolution of any further complaints.

Social insurance institutes establish their coverage policies based on their legal charters and determine the services and drugs provided, in this latter case based on approvals by the General Health Council and by COFEPRIS. The Social Insurance Law governing IMSS provides Mexico's president with the power to decree coverage of occupationally defined population groups, or to collaborate with the federal government in providing services on the basis of solidarity if so requested and if funds are provided in full by the federal government. The most recent population group covered by presidential decree was that of students of public universities in the 1980s. Services provided by IMSS on a solidarity basis are delivered through IMSS-Bienestar for the extreme poor who are identified through poverty indicators and funded directly by the Ministry of the Treasury on an annual basis.

■ **2.6.5** *Regulation and governance of payers*

Public payers and providers are vertically integrated within social insurance institutions and, to varying degrees, also within MoH-funded and operated services. In the case of the MoH, up until the demise of Seguro Popular part of its funding was managed by CNPSS at the federal level and by REPSS at the state level at arm's length from provision. Another part is still funded directly to providers, used mostly to pay for human resources. Private insurance comes in two forms: the first – indemnity insurance – is a more traditional private insurance model that covers the costs of health incurred and does not restrict choice of providers. The second – known as Specialized Health Insurance – is like managed care, where insurers contract with providers and insure the policy holders for the cost of care provided only by those in their network.

SOCIAL INSURANCE INSTITUTIONS

Social insurance institutions are self-funded according to their laws, pooling the contributions of various sources under a financing department. The federal government finances social insurance through line item 19 "Social Security contributions" according to the annual Federal Expenditure Budget (PEF) based on the expected number of people to be covered for the budget year. Specific laws for each fund determine the contribution by the government, employers and employees (see section 2.2.3), usually as a percentage of employee income or – in the case of some government contributions – as a fixed sum based on an official minimum wage.

Health benefits of social insurance institutions typically include workers' compensation and maternity and sickness insurance. Institutes prepare annual operational plans for each fund and allocate a budget to pay for the various line items accordingly. Institutes regulate the rights of beneficiaries with few exclusions, such as cosmetic surgery and prosthesis. Institutions specify a 2-month period of extension of benefits after employee cessation according to their own laws. IMSS insurance funds are independently audited annually and the reports are published to inform the federal executive and Congress on the institution's financial situation.

The financial imbalance between income and expenditure has been growing within IMSS and similarly challenges ISSSTE and other social insurance funds. IMSS law requires all of its new employees to be fully funded for their current costs and for their pension scheme. However, no regulations are yet in place to secure funding for older hires whose pension scheme is technically bankrupt, leading to an increasing proportion of current income being allocated to paying for the pensions of retiring employees.

FUNDING FOR THE NON-INSURED

The regulation of health care payers for the non-insured population is more complex given the number of contributors involved as well as the complex network of providers (see sections 2.2.1 and 2.2.2). Up until 2004, most funding was contributed by the federal government through the MoH via the Health Services Contribution Fund (FASSA). FASSA earmarks fiscal resources for health care for the non-insured in federal budget line item 33 "Federal contributions for federal states and municipalities" and is subject to full accountability by state governments. FASSA pays mostly for the historical budget for human resources and infrastructure maintenance.

With the introduction of the SPSS in 2004, resources were earmarked from federal budget line item 12 "MoH Administration" to pay for the services covered by Seguro Popular. Funding was channelled to CNPSS on a per beneficiary basis in three parts as prescribed in the General Health Law. The first is the social allocation (*cuota social*), estimated on the basis of a fixed 3.92% of a minimum wage. The second, a federal solidary contribution (ASF, *Aportación Solidaria Federal*) was estimated to be at least 1.5 times the social allocation. The third part consisted of a state government solidary contribution (ASE), which was set to be at least 0.5 of the *cuota social*. The federal contribution – ASF – is in turn allocated to CNPSS through two separate mechanisms. The first was calculated on the basis of past historical funding plus special federal programmes and commitments for the uninsured and is directly allocated to state health services and labelled as the "aligned" ASF. The second mechanism was allocated to CNPSS earmarked as "complementary" ASF for integration with the *cuota social* and the ASE. The CNPSS required the ASE to be delivered in at least 30% in cash to REPSS, while the remainder can be accounted for as investments or as direct state government expenditure in health.

The CNPSS established the annual SPSS budget on the basis of the number of estimated Seguro Popular beneficiaries. A continuous challenge faced by CNPSS was the inability to fully avoid simultaneous registration of individuals with both Seguro Popular and social insurance institutions, due mostly to the high levels of labour mobility and the delayed notification of CNPSS of new incorporations by IMSS (see section 7.3).

The MoH and the General Health Council were charged with identifying duplicate registries and ensuring CNPSS does not double fund for individuals also registered with IMSS. Double registration was only allowed in the case of seasonal workers with brief and transient protection by IMSS (González Block et al., 2018c).

The General Health Law specified the amounts of SPSS funding that was to be allocated to cover services included in the benefits package – the CAUSES list of essential interventions and medicines, as well as the high-cost interventions covered in the catastrophic expenditures fund (FPGC). After deducting a fixed percentage for administration, CNPSS transferred 89% of the funds to the states for CAUSES and retained 11% for direct payment for FPGC interventions. Since 2009, CNPSS set allocation quotas for CAUSES funds to ensure that at least 20% is spent on preventive interventions and not more than 40% on human resources and 30% on medicines.

All health care providers funded by SPSS had to be accredited by the MoH. Providers were accredited every 5 years to provide CAUSES or FPGC services. For CAUSES, providers needed to comply with general infrastructure and human resource requirements, while for FPGC, they must have accredited requirements for each specific intervention. Accreditation was the remit of the DGCES, while CNPSS supervised and inspected FPGC providers directly. The General Audit of the Federation (ASFed) audited REPSS and state authorities to ensure compliance with general financial rules.

A reform to the General Health Law was undertaken in 2014 to streamline SPSS funding in response to lack of transparency, delays and misallocation of resources and even fraud. Each REPSS was ordered to open accounts with the Federal Treasury to manage at least 50% of the CNPSS transfers. This reform thus avoided the allocation of cash to state treasuries and ensures more transparent disbursements, especially for the purchase of medicines at the federal level through consolidation with other public institutions.

The reform also established minimum time periods of 5 days for the funds allocated in cash to state administrators to be delivered to the REPSS, with the threat of penal sanctions for non-compliance.

The new Policy for Free Health Services and Medicines and INSABI have yet to establish funding and payment guidelines, which should be operational in 2020. It is expected that CAUSES and FPGC will be substituted with an integrated guideline set to promote integrated care and ensure full funding across treatment pathways. Coverage is expected to be gradually expanded, although it is uncertain if funding will be made available in sufficient amounts to attain universal coverage by the end of the current administration in 2024.

PRIVATE HEALTH INSURANCE

Private insurance companies provide indemnity insurance against health expenditures through reimbursing policy holders, hospitals or physicians. Indemnity insurance is subject to regulation by the National Insurance and Securities Commission (CNSF) to ensure they have the financial capacity to meet their contracted risks. Regulation imposes no limitations on policy benefits and insured sums and policies can be contracted on an individual or group basis. Indemnity insurance law reforms in 2015 now enable reimbursement for preventive services so long as they are not directly supplied by insurers.

Private insurers can also participate in Special Health Insurance Institutions (ISES), an insurance model that both reimburses health costs and provides preventive, curative and rehabilitation services directly through their own or contracted infrastructure. ISES were set up as a response to a requirement of the North American Free Trade Agreement to have a legal framework for managed care organizations in place for the early 2000s. The proposal met opposition in Congress from the IMSS trade union as ISES would compete for tripartite contributions. The compromise as reflected in the 1999 reform to the General Law of Institutions and Mutualist Insurance Societies was the creation of ISES without the obligation of IMSS to outsource medical care based on a capitated model. The law gave no incentives for managed care providers to operate in this market, leading to a slow, minimal growth of ISES and to low levels of regulation. In 2018, a total of 11 ISES were in operation, of which two were specialized in dentistry. Population covered totalled 120 000 people and some ISES were owned by banks and other firms, mostly those that have agreements with IMSS for the direct provision of services (DGCES, 2015) (see sections 2.1.5 and 2.2.3).

ISES are free to establish their own health plans and exemptions but must be qualified to provide a basic preventive and care package of medical or dental care subject to MoH approval. ISES are required by CNSF to name an independent medical supervisor to oversee compliance with programme utilization, the operation of the provider network, appropriate coverage, compliance with the General Health Law and Official Mexican Standards, and complaint follow-up. Comptrollers report quarterly to the CNSF and to the MoH and the MoH issues periodic re-accreditation.

■ **2.6.6** *Regulation and governance of providers*

Health care providers in Mexico are regulated and governed through social insurance and MoH institutions at the federal level. There is also some participation by professional and industry associations, in particular in the case of medical specialty councils that are responsible for issuing medical licenses (see section 4.2.1).

All MoH and private health facilities are regulated by COFEPRIS through licensing, surveillance and inspection while the General Health Council offers voluntary accreditation for hospitals. Social insurance institutions are responsible for their own regulation and may request accreditation from the GHC. Official Mexican Standards regulate each type of facility according to structural requirements and are in theory applicable to all health facilities. COFEPRIS carries out inspections in coordination with state health authorities, focusing mostly on private sector providers. DGCES, for its part, accredited MoH and private providers as a requirement to receive subsidies and payments from Seguro Popular.

Voluntary accreditation by the General Health Council is organized through the National System for Certification of Medical Care Establishments (SiNaCEAM), developed with the support of the Joint Commission International, a non-profit accreditation firm in the United States (see section 5.4.2 for hospital accreditation). SiNaCEAM evaluates the implementation of the "Patient Safety Model", which is based on international standards and has been enriched in response to the Mexican context (ANFEM, 2018). The General Health Council is now making plans to accredit all public providers, substituting the accreditation functions previously held by the federal MoH.

Hospitals are organized in two industry associations: the National Association of Private Hospitals (ANHP), representing 79 of the country's 94 larger-than-50-beds hospitals, and the Mexican Association of Hospitals (AMH), which represents both public and private hospitals but with an emphasis on public hospitals and a focus on training and social relations (Asociación Nacional de Hospitales Privados, 2018). No national association represents the 2829 private hospitals with fewer than 50 beds, although some medium-sized hospitals are organized in commercial associations, such as the Mexican Consortium of Hospitals, with close to 40 independent members.

General and specialist physicians are mostly organized at the state and national level through colleges, councils and associations with the main objective of ensuring professional development and accreditation. State colleges are confederated at the national level through the National College of Physicians. Membership in colleges and associations is low in the case of general physicians, with the National College of Physicians only having in the order of 15 000 members. Due to their requiring obligatory accreditation, specialty councils and associations have a wider membership. Labour relations are not the remit of these associations, which are regulated mostly through individual professional contracts or through employee contracts in the private sector, or through collective contracts in the public sector (see section 4.2.1).

■   **2.6.7** *Regulation of services and goods*

BASIC BENEFIT PACKAGE

Benefits packages vary across the coverage schemes. Social insurance institutes establish their own benefits packages; they are not explicitly defined, and there are a few exclusions; for example, cosmetic surgery and prosthesis. The benefits are broader than health coverage and also typically include pensions, maternity leave and other social services such as day care. The benefits package for Seguro Popular was explicitly defined and was less generous than the social insurance packages (see sections 3.2.2 and 3.3.1). With INSABI it is expected to attain similar, unrestricted packages across all public institutions.

HEALTH TECHNOLOGY ASSESSMENT

Health technology assessment is undertaken by MoH and each of the major social insurance institutions. The National Centre of Technological Excellence in Health (CENETEC) was established by MoH in 2004 as a deconcentrated, arm's-length MoH agency to manage and evaluate health technologies for all subsystems making up the NHS. Its focus is on economic evaluation, clinical guidelines, biomedical engineering and telehealth. Economic evaluation is also carried out by the General Health Council in the area of pharmaceuticals as the first authoritative step towards the inclusion of pharmaceuticals into the public sector. While social insurance institutions voluntarily accept their rulings, IMSS and ISSSTE also engage in some form of economic evaluation to determine final inclusion of pharmaceuticals and devices into their own lists.

CENETEC coordinates the development of clinical guidelines through the establishment of sectoral committees in collaboration with the most important health institutions and specialty councils, distributing topics across specific institutions who chair the development of each clinical guideline. CENETEC published 699 clinical guidelines for 2014, though there have been challenges with implementation. DGCES is responsible for implementing the guidelines, though the process is voluntary and varies widely across institutions in terms of the resources available and extent to which guidelines are adopted (Gutiérrez et al., 2015).

CENETEC is also responsible for analysing the cost–effectiveness of new, expensive technologies and for providing Certificates of Need for Medical Equipment, which are required by MoH and state-level health authorities prior to purchase. Certificates are granted by the General Directorate for Health Planning and Development (DGPLADES) according the Master Plan for Physical Infrastructure for Health (PMI).

■ **2.6.8** *Regulation and governance of pharmaceuticals*

GOVERNMENT REGULATION

COFEPRIS is the chief agency responsible for regulating pharmaceutical innovation, safety, efficacy, prescription and dispensation. The main governmental regulatory tools are product licensing and pharmacovigilance. The Ministry of Commerce coordinates voluntary price controls for the private sale of pharmaceuticals and the Federal Commission for Economic Competition (COFECE) regulates production and commercialization to ensure competitive markets.

A reform to the General Health Law in the 1990s promoted the introduction of generic medicines into the public sector and the private market. This reform established bioequivalence requirements and a later reform facilitated the participation of third-party laboratories to test prospective generics. COFEPRIS has prioritized the licensing of generic medicines, although COFECE established that a wide gap still exists for the penetration of generics into the Mexican market due to barriers to competition (Comisión Federal de Competencia Económica, 2017). From 2006, COFEPRIS markedly improved its licensing processes by decreasing approval time. COFEPRIS gained Level IV certification by the Pan American Health Organization (PAHO), which recognizes it as a regulator with the capacity to act as a regional centre of reference for pharmaceutical efficacy, safety and quality.

With respect to price controls of patent medicines, two mechanisms are in place for the public and private sector, respectively. CCPNMIS is the sole government mechanism that negotiates with patent holders the prices for public consumption on the basis of the approved institutional medicine lists. The commission was integrated in 2009 in response to the economic crisis by the Ministries of the Treasury and Budget, Commerce and the MoH, as well as by IMSS and ISSSTE, the Comptroller General and COFECE. CCPNMIS has specific committees to analyse reference pricing and cost–effectiveness and has steadily increased the number of drug price specifications included, with a total of 230 involving 46 laboratories (CCNPMIS, 2016).

Patent medicine price controls are established for the private sector through obligatory registration of maximum sale prices with the Ministry of Commerce and through mandatory package labelling. Laboratories voluntarily establish their maximum prices based on a Ministry of Commerce guideline that considers wholesale prices in countries with the highest sales and distribution as well as Mexico's particular dispensation costs. In 2017, the Ministry of Commerce published maximum prices for nearly 280 patented medicines (Secretaría de Comercio, 2017; Procuraduria Federal del Consumidor, 2006).

PHARMACEUTICAL SELF-REGULATION

Pharmaceutical self-governance is structured through the National Chamber of the Pharmaceutical Industry (Canifarma), the Mexican Association of Innovative Pharmaceutical Industry (AMIIF), which consists of mostly multinational pharma, and the Mexican Pharmaceutical Consortium (CFM). Ethical conduct is self-regulated through the Council for Ethics and Transparency of the Pharmaceutical Industry (CETIFARMA). As with other chambers, Canifarma had its origins as a government-controlled association to which all industrialists had to belong to do business in Mexico. Mandatory membership was abrogated in early 2000 and today Canifarma operates as a voluntarily association that serves as the main, although not exclusive, channel of representation with government. Canifarma incorporates most and certainly the largest pharma, medical and diagnostic devices, and reagents companies in Mexico, with close to 160 members, all of whom are also CETIFARMA members.

Among the most important Canifarma commissions are those for public provision, regulatory matters, research, innovation and technological development and safety. The public provision commission addresses issues emerging mostly from the bulk (consolidated) purchases undertaken by IMSS and recently also by the Ministry of the Treasury on behalf of most public institutions, and supports price reduction while limiting its negative consequences, such as the potential elimination of small players from the marketplace. Canifarma also supports government regulation through facilitating access to COFEPRIS for its members. Among the issues currently being explored by Canifarma is the introduction of risk-based purchasing agreements between the pharma innovation industry and the public sector, to facilitate market access for expensive innovative drugs based on value for health and not only on price. Challenges facing such agreements – as in other parts of the world – are the availability of information on health results and the complexity of administrative arrangements (Health Research Institute, 2017). Canifarma together with COFEPRIS were co-signatories in 2017 of the first agreement to facilitate research and innovation through closer working relationships between IMSS, CONACYT and AMIIF and its members, particularly to resolve the issues pertaining to economic benefits accruing from research across all the parties involved (Velázquez Ramírez, 2017).

The liberalization of industry associations and chambers led to the establishment of other industry consortia, most notably the Mexican Pharmaceutical Consortium (CFM). This consortium coordinates six large pharmaceutical companies that are distinguished by their innovation and export capacity. It aims to strengthen and expand the Mexican pharmaceutical industry through facilitating innovation, linkages to the production and service sectors and to promote quality and capitalization. The National Association of Pharmaceutical Manufacturers (ANAFAM) coordinates some of the largest national generic drug manufacturers in the country, while the Mexican Association of Interchangeable Generic Medicines (AMEGI) groups the largest multinational generic drug manufacturers.

■ 2.7 **Person-centred care**

Patient empowerment in Mexico has been pursued indirectly as a matter of labour rights since the Constitution of 1917 and more directly through the amendment to the Constitution in 1983 that established the right to health protection. In this last development, the government is charged with ensuring that all people have access to health services according to needs, although differences persist given the segmentation of the health system (see sections 2.2.1 and 2.5.1). Beginning in 2003, the General Health Law specified patient rights for the beneficiaries of the Seguro Popular, but did not extend to social insurance beneficiaries or private sector clients. The MoH supports the arbitration of complaints through the National Commission for Medical Arbitration (CONAMED) while the National Commission for Human Rights (CNDH) intervenes in selected high-profile cases. A Patient's Charter was published by CONAMED and replicated in human rights guidelines by the Ministry of the Interior, consisting of a 10-point list of broad patient rights.

2.7.1 *Patient information*

There are no dedicated databases or information outlets specialized in providing patients with information regarding Mexico's health system actors and functions. The most important source of patient information is the National Health and Nutrition Survey, undertaken every 5 years since 1995. The National Institute of Public Health facilitates access to the database and disseminates reports with aggregate data on health needs and health service demand at state and national levels. IMSS, ISSSTE provide call centres for patient orientation and to make appointments for primary care. Seguro Popular provided similar information services, which are expected to be carried forward by INSABI. In most cases, institutional websites provide health promotion information and facilitate health service access. There is limited information on quality and costs of care in the private sector, in spite of the high levels of out-of-pocket expenditure.

There have been periodic calls for the establishment of a national information centre on health provider performance and costs across the public and private sectors, which would aim to inform patient choice to spur competitiveness, reduce prices and, ultimately, improve quality. As yet, no concrete results have been achieved.

2.7.2 *Patient choice*

Patients covered by social insurance or by public coverage are generally assigned medical facilities and family or general physicians without having any choice. Assigned doctors can only be changed on account of complaints and following bureaucratic procedures. Medicines are dispensed through pharmacies within institutions, and when there are shortages, patients usually access these medicines out-of-pocket in private pharmacies. In 2013, complaints about IMSS led to a proposal to redress drug shortages through issuing vouchers for provision within private pharmacies. However, the response was limited to using IMSS pharmacies with guaranteed supplies, which required patients to travel beyond their neighbourhoods and clinics. Rather than empowering patients, IMSS has focused on improving quality through administrative procedures, such as reducing waiting times through eliminating the fixed doctor allocation and allowing patients to be seen by any doctor in the clinic based on a queuing system.

2.7.3 *Patient rights*

Rights to receive the services outlined in the benefits package were specified in the General Health Law for those covered by Seguro Popular (funded through SPSS) (see Table 2.3). Rights were monitored by CNPSS by ensuring purchasing of drugs, certification of facilities and facilitating complaints through a national call centre and complaints boxes at the facility level. Compliance with patient rights was supervised by specialized medical managers (*gestores médicos*), employed by Seguro Popular in hospitals and primary care facilities. These managers were also in charge of establishing eligibility for free care according to the funded interventions' lists. The General Health Law now mandates universal coverage of all services through INSABI, although it is not clear how these rights will be supervised. Indeed, health managers were the first component of Seguro Popular to disappear in early 2019.

Social insurance institutions are governed by boards made up of employer, employee and federal government representatives. However, employee rights are only weakly enforced as employee representatives within IMSS are appointed only at the highest levels and by trade union confederations that do not represent the IMSS beneficiary base. Indeed, only 3% of IMSS beneficiaries belong to confederations, and only 6% are unionized (see section 2.2.3). Furthermore, the remit of governing employer and employee unions participating in IMSS governance through the technical council are to reconcile their interests and not to ensure health as such. Instead, most of the governance agenda has to do with the appointment of directors and with financial and administrative matters. A very small proportion of the agenda addresses specific health issues and not much addresses health complaints (González Block, 2018). In the case of the small number of trade-unionized beneficiaries, patient complaints may be taken to local trade union representatives for consideration by health providers.

TABLE 2.3 Situation of patient rights in Mexico

SITUATION	Y/N	COMMENTS
Protection of patient rights		
Does a formal definition of patient rights exist at national level?	Y	The only explicit health-related right at the national level is the constitutional right to health protection. The Constitution recognizes the right to health of the 1967 International Covenant on Economic, Social and Cultural Rights.
Are patient rights included in specific legislation or in more than one law?	Y	Patient rights were only protected for SPSS (Seguro Popular) beneficiaries through a set of 15 rights defined in the General Health Law, which disappeared with the INSABI reform in 2019. The MoH published a 10-point guideline of patient rights.
Does the legislation conform with WHO's patient rights framework?	Y	In so far as the Constitution recognizes the International Covenant, specifying the right to health as the right of everyone to the enjoyment of the highest attainable standard of physical and mental health.
Patient complaints avenues		
Are hospitals required to have a designated desk responsible for collecting and resolving patient complaints?	N	Only hospitals funded by SPSS were required to have a complaints box, not a desk. Social insurance institutions have of their own accord established complaints offices, although they are not specific to health issues. Specific procedures are applied to ensure that complaints are reviewed and addressed.
Is a health-specific ombudsman responsible for investigating and resolving patient complaints about health services?	Y	The National Commission for Medical Arbitration (CONAMED) is responsible for investigation, although it has limited powers to do so and its resolutions are not binding.
Other complaint avenues?	Y	The National Commission for Human Rights takes charge of prominent human rights violations related to health.
Liability/compensation		
Is liability insurance required for physicians and/or other medical professionals?	N	
Can legal redress be sought through the courts in the case of medical error?	Y	However, very few cases are actually pursued.

Source: Authors

■ **2.7.4** *Complaints procedures*

General complaints against personnel or processes within public institutions are channelled through Organs for Internal Control (OIC), which report to the Ministry of the Public Function – the general comptroller. OIC can be reached through its website, an 800 number, or in person by visiting their general offices in Mexico City. Complaints can also be lodged with health facility user orientation offices or complaints units within state offices or at the national level, while internal guidelines establish that all complaints – no matter how they are lodged – should be considered.

In the case of IMSS, complaint resolutions must be first resolved by employer–employee complaint committees established by the technical council at the national level or by state councils or councils established in each high specialty hospital. Within state-level MoH facilities, written complaints are analysed jointly by the OIC and the health authority.

Civil medical malpractice complaints lodged with the MoH at federal or state levels as well as against private providers or complaints not resolved by IMSS or ISSSTE are taken up by CONAMED. CONAMED addresses around 90% of complaints by reorienting patients on a fast track. Cases not resolved at this stage are admitted for conciliation through technical analyses. Around 48% of these complaints are resolved through conciliation, 2.5% sent for arbitration and the rest remain unresolved.

CONAMED resolutions are not binding and if complaints are not resolved they must be taken to the courts. Orientation by CONAMED is limited in the case of IMSS to reviewing the written complaint submitted by patients. IMSS centralizes all conciliation and arbitration processes in Mexico City and responds in writing to both CONAMED and the patient with regard to its resolutions. Over half of complaints lodged with CONAMED are from IMSS patients and delays often go beyond the 2-year period allocated to such cases. Many complaints involving the private sector are not resolved due to an unwillingness to proceed by either party into the conciliation or arbitration stages (Fajardo Dolci, 2014).

■ **2.7.5** *Patients and cross-border health care**

Mexico supplies a large body of migrant workers to the United States and Canada, with 11.9 million Mexican migrants residing in the USA in 2016 (Aldana & Reyes, 2019). Between 2009 and 2014, Mexico sent close to 1 million immigrants per year to the USA. Net migration is closer today to 0 given the number of migrants returning to Mexico. Yet an estimated 31.5% (3.8 million) of Mexicans living in the United States do not have health insurance, with even fewer (30%) of those who have lived in the United States for more than 10 years having health insurance (Aldana & Reyes, 2019). Therefore, many of the Mexicans living in the United States access health care in Mexico and pay out of pocket.

Migrant workers coming to Mexico from Central America have to pay out of pocket to access public and private health facilities, except those interventions that are universally provided for free such as immunizations and family planning. However, the López Obrador administration has promised to provide these migrants with full access to services on a par with the Mexican uninsured.

Migrants tend to satisfy their health needs while traversing Mexico on their way to the United States or when working in Mexico, mostly in the southern states. Given the high costs of medical care in the USA, Mexico's northern border has become a hub for medical care and the sale of pharmaceuticals for US residents living in bordering states. Migrants use a variety of strategies to compensate for their lack of health insurance and access to health services in the United States, including self-medication, home remedies, telephone consultation in Mexico, travel to border towns to obtain care, returning to their places of origin in Mexico, and regular medical care during their visits to Mexico (Vega 2019). The mental health situation of migrants from Central American countries crossing Mexico to the United States is of concern given the highly stressful situations they face, including sexual violence. Studies suggest these populations face ailments related to stress, anxiety and extreme suffering, though with low levels of demand and supply of mental health services (Temores Alcantara et al., 2015).

---

* Dr Nelly Salgado and Dr Fernando Riosmena are acknowledged for their contributions to this section, based on Salgado et al. (in press).

CROSS-BORDER HEALTH POLICY

In 1943, at the request of the US Public Health Service, PAHO set up a field office at the El Paso, Texas border. That same year, the US–Mexico Border Health Association (USMBHA) was established as a non-profit organization aimed at promoting the development of transnational public health organizations and practises in the border area (Collins-Dogrul, 2006). While the PAHO office has since disappeared, together with USMBHA it contributed to the establishment of effective mechanisms not only for exchanging information, resources and ideas, but also for developing projects in collaboration with professionals from both countries.

The government of Mexico has, since 1990, made some effort to support health services for migrants in the USA and on their return trips. IMSS established the Migrant Programme whereby farm worker unions, in agreement with the Mexican government, offered migrants and their families coverage to IMSS' Family Health Insurance in Mexico. Yet, the programme failed to achieve full-scale implementation at the time, due partly to the low priority that IMSS assigned to expanding voluntary coverage (Collins-Dogrul, 2006). Since 2010, the Mexican government promoted Seguro Popular registration in United States consulates for Mexican citizens residing there as a means of ensuring their health coverage upon return to Mexico.

After the passage of NAFTA in 1994, concerns mounted over border health issues, culminating in the creation in 2000 of the US–Mexico Border Health Commission. The commission's 26 members include public health officials and professionals from the 10 bordering states, the ministers of health from both federal governments and, in the case of Mexico, state-level ministers of health (Comisión de Salud Fronteriza México-Estados Unidos, 2017). Between 2000 and 2010, the commission addressed the most prevalent border health needs, on one hand, by organizing a Binational Health Week, the National Infant Immunization/Vaccination Week in the Americas, and the US–Mexico Binational Infectious Disease Conference; and on the other, by setting up the Binational Border Health Research Work Group and Expert Panel.

Since 2001, the federal Mexican Health Promotion Directorship, has been operating the programme Leave Healthy, Return Healthy (VSRS; *Vete Sano Regresa Sano*) throughout Mexico, with the purpose of educating migrants about the need to increase their resilience to the severe conditions, social isolation and lifestyle changes imposed by migration. VSRS disseminates information on lifestyle changes and contingencies common to the migration process as well as the health risks to be expected in transit and upon destination. It is particularly active at health fairs during the winter months; that is, when migrants visit their communities of origin. VSRS coordinates its activities with other Mexican immigration and health offices at the state level and the Binational Health Week organizing committee (Secretaría de Salud, 2007a).

The MoH and the Ministry of Foreign Affairs installed health information booths (*Ventanillas de Salud*, VdS) in 50 Mexican consulates throughout the United States, to promote health and community outreach through agreements with local NGOs (Secretaría de Relaciones Exteriores, 2016). Care for migrant children that arrived in the USA unaccompanied and that are repatriated to Mexico, as well as for repatriated adults, have been a high priority in the six northern Mexican border states. The Ministry of Foreign Affairs implements the Repatriation Programme for Seriously Ill Nationals, funded by both ministries but mainly by the migrants with their own resources. Predominant diagnoses include chronic renal failure, brain disease, paraplegia, cancer and mental illness.

CROSS-BORDER HEALTH SERVICES UTILIZATION

Utilization of Mexican health services by US residents is driven by their being of acceptable quality at low cost, with more care offered that factors in their own language and other cultural considerations (Landeck and Garza, 2002; Wallace et al., 2009). In the early 2000s, over 41% of *Latino* households in Laredo, Texas, were estimated to utilize medical services in Mexico while up to 250 000 health-related crossings were reported per month in Tijuana, at the California–Mexico border (de Guzmán et al., 2007). Up to 1.2% of public hospital discharges at the Mexican border are offered to in-transit migrants primarily for injuries, while private hospitals report elective surgeries as their chief causes of admission, followed by diabetes and other chronic diseases. Mexican migrants living in the USA tend to access medical services in Mexico while visiting their communities of origin, partly due to their lack of health insurance in the USA, as well as their low acculturation, inability to afford care in the USA, and high medical costs (Aldana & Reyes, 2019;

Vega, 2019). Up to 20% of hospital services required in 2008 by migrants who keep in touch with economically dependent relations in Mexico were obtained in their communities of origin (González Block & de la Sierra de la Vega, 2011). Repatriated migrants are admitted to hospitals mostly due to chronic renal failure, brain damage and mental illness, and correspond to about 1% of discharges from MoH hospitals in high- and very-high-migration municipalities.

Migrants in the USA tend to send money to relatives back home, which may be used to pay for health care. A survey at the Mexican consulate in Los Angeles in 2010 suggested that at least 25% of the money received from migrants is spent on health care in Mexico, while a study of health expenditure in Mexican households with migrant family members suggested that up to 32% of remittances are spent on health care (González Block et al., 2012; Amuedo Dorantes et al., 2007). Based on total remittances received, household health care spending was projected at US$ 7.8 billion, equivalent to 0.98% of GDP in 2007, one sixth of the overall health care expenditure and one third of private out-of-pocket spending for health care.

3

Financing

■ Chapter summary

- Total health expenditure in Mexico has increased significantly since 2000 to 5.7% of GDP in 2015, which is lower than the Latin America and Caribbean average and considerably lower than the OECD average.
- Public spending on health has also increased since 2000, but still remains relatively low, at about 54% of total health spending, with a significant role for out-of-pocket payments, at 42% of total spending.
- Social insurance is financed from employee and employer contributions, and government subsidies. In 2015, about 30% of total health expenditure was from social insurance, which covered 42% of the population.
- Public coverage for those without social insurance was provided up until 2019 through Seguro Popular, a programme funded mostly through the federal budget according to the SPSS; making up 24% of total health expenditure in 2015.
- Private insurance plays a small but growing role in funding health care in Mexico; making up 5% of total health expenditure in 2015 up from 2.3% in 2000.
- Provider payment models are heterogeneous across payers and providers. The dominant payment model among federal and state governments, and social insurance institutions, is a historical budget.

◼ 3.1 **Health expenditure**

Total health expenditure in Mexico in 2015 was 1062 billion Mexican pesos, equivalent to US$ 1008.7 billion PPP and 5.7% of GDP, according to the national health accounts (Table 3.1). The average annual growth rate for total health expenditure was higher than the GDP growth rate. However, there has been a slowdown in the growth of health spending, falling from 8.5% per year between 2001 and 2005, to 4.2% between 2006 and 2010, and to 2.6% between 2011 and 2015. According to 2015 World

FIG. 3.1 Total health expenditures as a share (%) of GDP in OECD countries, 2018

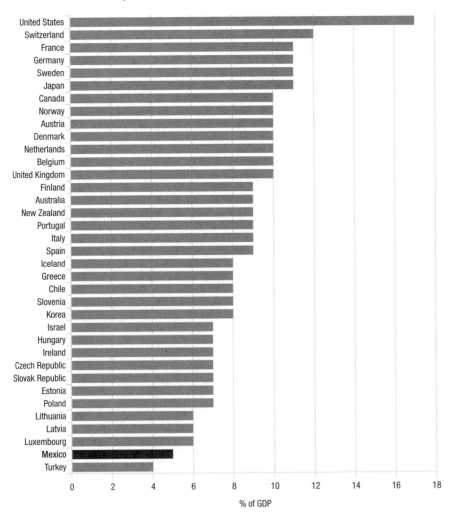

Source: OECD (2019)

Bank estimates,* the proportion of GDP destined for health in Mexico was 5.9%, an estimate that followed historical financing trends and was higher than the figure reported by national health accounts (5.7%; Table 3.1). This figure is lower than that registered in other Latin American and Caribbean countries such as Argentina (6.8%), Chile (8.1%) and Brazil (8.9%). According to the OECD, spending on health in Mexico was 5.7% of GDP compared with the OECD average of 8.8% in 2018 (Figure 3.1).

From 2005 to 2015, growth in health expenditure was very low, maintaining health spending at around 5.9% of GDP (Figure 3.2). Thus, as of 2005, Mexico has consistently had the lowest level of health spending as a proportion of GDP in the group of countries with similar or higher levels of development in the Americas, such as Argentina, Brazil, Canada, Chile, Costa Rica and USA.

---

* Differences between World Bank and OECD estimates are due to the nature of the data. OECD estimates are based on the System of Health Accounts, which compiles expenditure data on a yearly basis from national health information systems. On the other hand, World Bank data is generated using time trend estimations on financing data. For this study, World Bank data is used to compare Mexico with other Latin American countries, while OECD estimates are used to compare North America and other OECD countries.

FIG. 3.2 Trends in health spending as a share (%) of GDP in Mexico and selected countries, 2000–2015

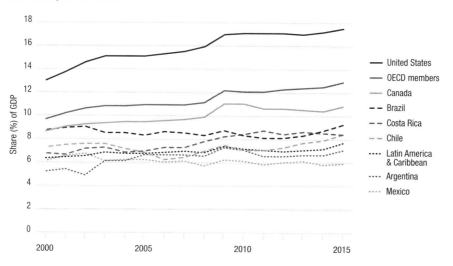

Sources: World Bank (2018), DGIS (2015b)

In terms of health expenditure per capita, in 2015 Mexico spent US$ 1009 PPP per capita (Table 3.1). Per capita health spending in Mexico was slightly lower than the average spent in Latin American and Caribbean countries (US$ 1081) (World Bank, 2018). Health spending per capita grew at a steady pace between 2000 and 2013, going from US$ 480.50 to US$ 1001.30 PPP (Table 3.1). In 2014, there was a drop in spending that was later overcome in 2015. It is worth mentioning that between 2000 and 2015, per capita spending doubled in real terms. According to OECD estimates, per capita spending in Mexico in 2018 was US$ 1138 (Figure 3.3), which was nearly one quarter of the OECD average (US$ 3992).

FIG. 3.3 Total health expenditures in US$ PPP per capita in OECD countries, 2018

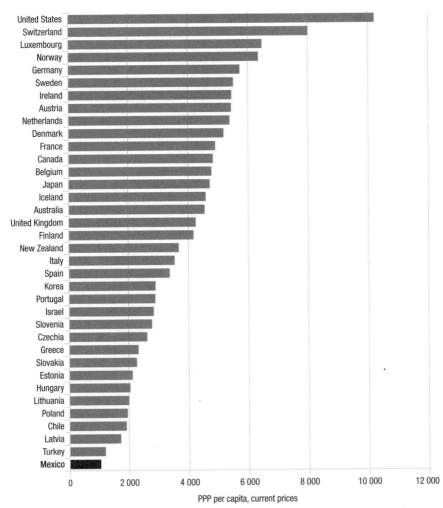

PPP per capita, current prices

Source: OECD (2019)

TABLE 3.1 Trends in health expenditure in Mexico, 2000–2015

INDICATOR	2000	2005	2010	2013	2015
Total expenditure on health care					
In current US$ PPP per capita	480.50	721.90	887.80	1001.30	1008.70
As share of GDP (%)[a]	5.9	6.0	5.9	5.9	5.7
Public expenditure on health care					
As share of total expenditure on health care (%)	43.7	43.4	52.0	54.6	53.8
As share of GDP (%)[a]	2.6	2.6	3.1	3.2	3.1
General government financing arrangements (for voluntary public coverage for uninsured) (% of total health expenditure)		16.6	22.1	23.5	24.2
Social insurance (statutory coverage for employed)		26.8	27.4	30.1	28.8
Private expenditure on health					
As share of total expenditure on health care (%)	56.3	56.6	48.0	45.4	46.2
As share of GDP (%)[a]	3.3	3.4	2.8	2.7	2.6
Out-of-pocket payments for health					
As share of total expenditure on health care (%)[a]	53.9	53.5	43.8	41.0	41.3
As share of private expenditure on health care (%)[a]	95.8	94.5	91.4	90.3	89.4
Voluntary private health insurance					
As share of total expenditure on health care (%)[a]	2.3	3.1	4.1	4.4	4.9
As share of private expenditure on health care (%)[a]	4.2	5.5	8.6	9.7	10.6
	2001–05	**2006–10**	**2011–15**		
Mean annual real growth rate in total health expenditurea	8.5	4.2	2.6		
Mean annual real growth rate in GDP	0.3	0.0	−0.6		

[a]DGIS (2015b)
Source: World Bank (2018)

Public expenditure on health, which includes government expenditure for the uninsured population and contributions to social insurance, increased from 43.7% in 2000 to 53.8% in 2015. This increase was a direct result of the 2003 reform of the General Health Law, which led to the implementation and continued expansion of the SPSS. With this system, and up until its demise in 2020, 43.5% of the population was covered by an alternative form of public financial protection and was thus financially protected from a limited set of high-cost interventions and, in theory, from most day-to-day health costs (see section 2.1.9). Currently, the proportion of total health expenditure that comes from the public sector is 51.6%, higher than Brazil (42.8%) and the Latin America and Caribbean average (51.7%), but lower than Costa Rica (76.0%), Argentina (71.4%) and Chile (60.8%), as well as being the lowest among all OECD countries (Figure 3.4). As shown in Figure 3.5, public spending on health in Mexico also makes up a slightly smaller share of total government spending than most other OECD countries, at about 10.4% compared with the OECD average of 24.5%.

The General Health Reform of 2003 redistributed health spending and led to a significant reduction in out-of-pocket spending, from 53.9% of total health expenditure in 2000 to 41.7% in 2015. On the other hand, private spending as a proportion of GDP decreased as of 2010, partly due to the global economic crisis but also the expansion of Seguro Popular and the reduction in the prices of private consultations and generic medicines. The proportion of total health expenditure that was from voluntary health insurance grew continuously from 2000 to 2015, doubling its share from 2.3% to 5.0% (Table 3.1).

Public spending on outpatient medical care in 2015 made up almost half of public health expenditure (47.1%) and represents one quarter (28.6%) of total health expenditure (Table 3.2). Public expenditure for hospitalization was 35.4% of public spending on health, while it represented 18.5% of total health expenditure. On the other hand, as a percentage of health spending, spending on drugs, pharmaceuticals and other laboratory supplies decreased between 2010 and 2015, from 15.1% to 14.5% (Table 3.3). Likewise, capital spending on medical facilities, which had been a policy promoted with the creation of the SPSS, was reduced by half between 2010 and 2015, from 5.1% to 2.7%.

FIG. 3.4 Public expenditure on health as a share (%) of current health expenditure in OECD countries, 2018

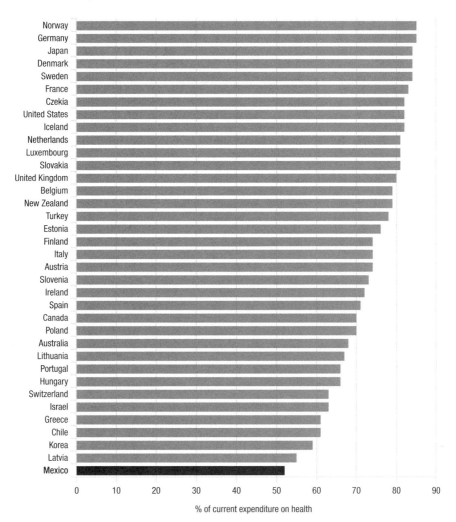

% of current expenditure on health

Source: OECD (2019)

FIG. 3.5 Public expenditure on health as a share (%) of government expenditure in OECD countries, 2018 or latest available data

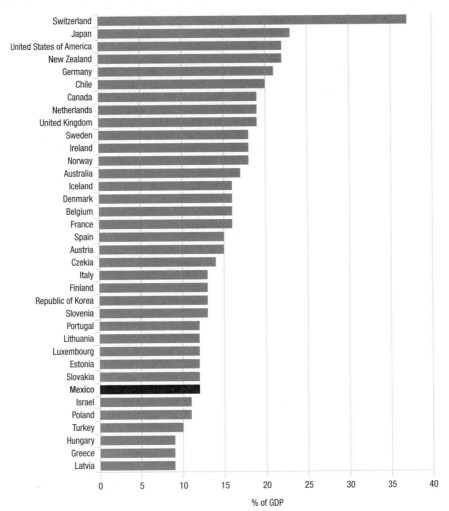

% of GDP

Source: World Bank (2018)

TABLE 3.2 Percentage distribution of total expenditure on health by health function and financing scheme, 2015

	PUBLIC SECTOR			PRIVATE SECTOR			
	TOTAL	GOVERNMENT SCHEMES	SOCIAL INSURANCE	TOTAL	VOLUNTARY HEALTH CARE PAYMENT SCHEMES	OUT-OF-POCKET PAYMENTS	TOTAL HEALTH EXPENDITURE
Health administration	9.2	9.5	8.9	18.0	18.0	0.0	6.0
Medical goods[a]	0.0	0.0	0.0	87.9	17.1	70.8	30.3
Public health	6.6	10.1	3.7	0.0	0.0	0.0	3.5
Medical services							
Hospital care	35.4	52.6	21.0	68.4	59.5	9.0	26.1
Outpatient medical services	47.1	26.1	64.8	11.3	2.0	9.3	28.6
Outpatient dental services	0.6	0.3	0.8	6.8	0.1	6.8	3.1
Home-based care services	0.0	0.0	0.0	0.5	0.1	0.5	0.2
Ancillary services	1.1	1.4	0.8	6.9	3.3	3.7	2.3

[a]Medical goods include drugs, pharmaceuticals, and other laboratory supplies

Source: MoH, OECD (2018b), spending matrices

TABLE 3.3 Public health expenditure on health by service input, 2010 and 2015 (%)

SERVICE INPUT	2010	2015
Drugs, pharmaceuticals and other lab supplies	15.1	14.5
Capital investment in medical facilities	5.1	2.7
Human resources	54.5	52.7
Services (utilities)	8.2	9.7
Other	17.2	20.4

Source: DGIS (2015a)

3.2 **Sources of revenue and financing flows**

The segmentation of the health system implies a complex financing architecture. The main source of health financing in Mexico is out-of-pocket spending, which represented 41.3% in 2015 (Table 3.1). In 2016, at least 104.4 million Mexicans (85.4% of population) had some type of health insurance coverage, either through employer-based social insurance, voluntary public coverage (Seguro Popular) or voluntary private insurance (González Block et al., 2018b) (see sections 2.2.3 and 2.2.4).

3.2.1 *Sources of revenue*

The intricate Mexican system of financing health is largely based on a person's ability to pay and their employment. Social insurance covers only workers in the formal private sector (IMSS), and those who work for the government (ISSSTE), the armed forces (Secretariat of National Defence (SEDENA) and Secretariat of the Navy (SEMAR)) and parastatals, such as PEMEX (Gómez Dantés et al., 2011) (see section 2.2.3). Its financing is tripartite, consisting of contributions from workers, employers and the government (Diario Oficial de la Federación, 1995; 2007). While contributions from employers and workers flow directly to IMSS, the government finances the institution via Branch 19 of the Federal Expenditure Budget (PEF). Currently, 28.8% of total health expenditure is from tripartite contributions to social insurance (Table 3.1) which covers 42.2% of the population (Figure 3.7).

Public services for members of the population without social insurance are provided through the federal and state governments and are mainly financed by general taxes and other government revenues, and to a lesser extent based on user fees paid out-of-pocket or, up until its demise, by annual contributions to Seguro Popular by households in deciles V to X of income. However, most affiliates in these income groups were enrolled without enforcing contributions (González Block et al., 2016). The federal monies are distributed through two funds: FASSA line item 33 of PEF, commonly called Federal Contributions, and line item 12, directed to administrative expenses but also to the payment of the SPSS' social fee (see sections 2.2.1 and 2.2.2).

After the 2003 reform of the General Health Law, the SPSS was created to expand health services and provide financial protection to the uninsured population, especially the poor. The structure of this financial protection scheme sought to emulate the tripartite contribution of social insurance, with contributions from households (according to capacity to pay), solidarity contributions from state governments and contributions from the federal government (federal contributions and line item 12) (Figure 3.6). In 2006, the New Generation Medical Insurance programme was introduced by presidential mandate, which later became the 21st Century Medical Insurance programme, aimed at covering all health needs not covered by the Seguro Popular for children under 5 years old. Government spending for the uninsured represented 24.2% of total health expenditure in 2015 (Table 3.1). Just under half of the financing (46.2%) in health is funded from private sources. In 2015, private insurance accounted for 4.9% of total health expenditure, a figure that more than doubled that estimated in 2000. The presence of private insurance in Mexico is small, although it has been gaining influence over time. According to recent estimates, 7.8% of the population has private insurance, mainly for major medical expenses (González Block et al., 2018b) (see section 2.2.4).

The Mexican population tends to use private services paid through out-of-pocket expenses even when they are insured. This is due to supply restrictions, the perception of poor quality, long waiting times for public services and, to a lesser extent, the costs caused by the high deductibles of private insurance.

As previously mentioned, the reform to the General Health Law and the creation of INSABI are leading to modifications of financial flows in ways that are still uncertain.

■ **3.2.2** *Financial flows*

The financial flows originate from contributions of companies and households to both government (as taxes) and social insurance institutions (as contributions) (Figure 3.6). The resources go through different financing schemes and are assigned to different providers for the purpose of covering differentiated groups of the population.

■ 3.3 **Overview of the statutory financing system**

The country's public contributory financing system is composed of several social insurance institutions (IMSS, ISSSTE and others), as well as SPSS components (Figure 3.6). Each body officially covers a different population and provides most of their services without user fees. Figure 3.7 describes these subsystems in terms of coverage, fundraising and pooling mechanisms.

FIG. 3.6 Financial flows for the payment of health providers, 2020

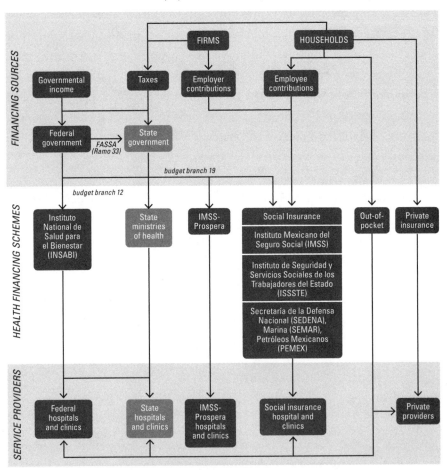

FASSA: Contribution Fund for Health Services; GHE: Governmental health expenditure plus user fees paid by households to public providers

Notes: Government budget is allocated among different funds (*Ramos*)

Source: Modified from González Block et al. (2018a)

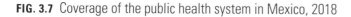

FIG. 3.7 Coverage of the public health system in Mexico, 2018

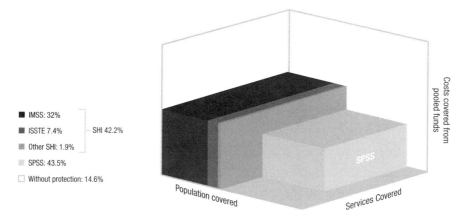

- ■ IMSS: 32%
- ■ ISSTE 7.4% ⎤
- ■ Other SHI: 1.9% ⎦ SHI 42.2%
- ▨ SPSS: 43.5%
- ☐ Without protection: 14.6%

SHI: Social Health Insurance
Source: Authors, based on Busse, Schreyögg & Gericke (2007);
Robert, Hsiao & Reich (2015); González-Block et al. (2018b)

■ 3.3.1 *Coverage*

SOCIAL INSURANCE

Social insurance institutions covered 42.2% of the total population in 2018. The largest social insurance institutions are IMSS, covering 33% of the population, and ISSSTE, which covers 7.4%. Social Insurance Law governing IMSS establishes that workers have the right to a range of insurance, as described in section 2.3.2. It should be added that IMSS, as with ISSSTE, offers two regimes: compulsory and voluntary. The compulsory scheme covers salaried workers, who by obligation are registered by their employers. Membership in the compulsory regime includes family members (spouses and/or cohabitants and children) of the worker, but ceases at the time the job is lost at which time the person and the employer no longer contribute. According to IMSS reports, 67.8% of the insured belong to this regime (IMSS, 2017). The voluntary scheme covering the remainder of the insured is open to non-salaried and farm workers as well as students (Diario Oficial de la Federación, 1995 and 2007; CNPSS, 2013).

SYSTEM FOR SOCIAL PROTECTION IN HEALTH

The SPSS, up until its demise in 2020, funded Seguro Popular to provide financial protection to those outside social insurance due to their employment as independent workers and inability to voluntarily enrol in IMSS, or who work for firms that have not registered with IMSS (see section 2.2.3). It covered 43.5% of the population, including beneficiaries of social programmes directed to rural areas or informal sector workers, the low-income population not benefiting from social programmes, and people who wish to join freely but who demonstrate that they do not have protection from other forms of insurance. Seguro Popular was free for beneficiaries in income deciles I to V (which includes the vast majority of Mexicans), while those in higher-income deciles paid an income-dependent yearly contribution.

The SPSS guaranteed its members access to a package of benefits free at the point-of-use, and the services included are listed in the CAUSES and on the FPGC list (see sections 2.2.1 and 2.2.2). CAUSES was composed of 294 interventions, which were classified into five groups: 1) prevention and health promotion (77 interventions, including vaccination and timely detection of diseases); 2) general and specialty medicine (120 interventions, including the screening of coverage pathologies of the Catastrophic Expenses Protection Fund and 21st Century Medical Insurance); 3) emergencies (69 interventions); 4) general surgery (54 interventions); and 5) obstetrics (24 interventions) (CNPSS, 2018b). Every 2 years, CNPSS decides what interventions are included in CAUSES.

Interventions covered by FPGC were determined through a consultative process led by the General Health Council applying criteria based on cost–effectiveness, affordability, financial protection, scientific expertise, supply and demand and social acceptance. The General Health Council submitted the list of selected interventions to the FPGC's technical committee, who decided on the services to be included and the costs to be covered depending on the availability of financial resources in the escrow (Official Gazette of the Federation, 2017c). As mentioned above, the FPGC covered 66 high-cost interventions (see section 2.1.9).

■ **3.3.2** *Collection and pooling*

Collection of funds varies according to public institutions and private insurance provider. Seguro Popular was funded mostly through federal and state taxes, with contributions by affiliates collected through the state ministries of health. IMSS and ISSSTE establish through their own laws the direct collection of contributions from employers and employees, with the federal government matching contributions. Employers are mandated to deduct employee contributions from paychecks. Government funds are allocated to each institution out of tax contributions. Other social insurance institutes such as those attached to PEMEX, SEDENA, SEMAR and the state employee institutes are fully funded directly from their budgets. Pooling of funds is limited within each of the social insurance institutions and the government programmes.

■ **3.3.3** *Purchasing and purchaser–provider relations*

SOCIAL INSURANCE

Social insurance institutions integrate purchasing and provision of health services; health services are purchased from providers they own, organized according to the level of complexity of care. Payment to these providers is made through programmatic budgets subject to care goals. Budgets are calculated based on historical spending patterns, and not on formulae of need, leading to maldistribution. To increase hospital spending efficiency, the payment method of Diagnostic Related Groups (DRGs) was attempted without success in both IMSS and ISSSTE.

When care cannot be provided in social insurance facilities directly, this care is purchased by contract with private providers or other public providers with authorization. This authorization is approved by a medical board, based on criteria of cost and investment capacity. An example of this type of service is haemodialysis for patients with chronic kidney disease. Social insurance institutions also contract services in the operating room, laparoscopy and hemodynamic, among others, where private companies specialized in service integration provide equipment and consumables as well as technical support for their operation, while the institutions provide medical and nursing staff.

These services are paid based on formulae that include the amount of services provided and the quality of care (user satisfaction) (González Block, 2018b).

SYSTEM FOR SOCIAL PROTECTION IN HEALTH (UNTIL 2019)

The SPSS purchased services from MoH hospitals, state health services and IMSS-Bienestar as well as from private providers. Funds are allocated under various mechanisms, including mainly collaboration agreements aligned to the achievement of goals, payment per case and to a lesser extent capitation (in a single case for primary care by a private provider in the state of Hidalgo). Fund 12 assigned via the Social Quota and the complementary federal solidarity contribution (ASF) is restricted to supplies, medicines, improvements in infrastructure and human resources in contact with the patient (see section 2.2.1). These human resources were contracted with a mix of service contracts and permanent unionized contracts, in accordance with the negotiation policies. The hiring of permanent positions has led the CNPSS to lose flexibility in the financial allocation, with the tendency that Seguro Popular spending becomes a historical expense (González Block, 2017).

The aligned ASF was assigned through FASSA (Fund 13) resources and distributed among federal entities through an allocation formula that is based on the infrastructure capacity of each federal entity and its needs. However, in practice, FASSA was – and will continue to be – allocated as a historical budget.

The design of the SPSS did not restrict – as do the social insurance institutions – the hiring of private providers and services. However, in practice, the same rules were followed as for social insurance, taking care not to affect the union interests of permanent workers. Private providers were only contracted in case services cannot be expanded on the basis of existing public infrastructure.

■ 3.4 Out-of-pocket health expenses

At the beginning of the 21st century, 56.3% of health spending was financed by private sources, mainly out-of-pocket (Table 3.1 and section 3.3). The majority of out-of-pocket spending would be classified as direct payments, as these are payments made for services that are not provided by statutory health coverage programmes or that are outside services covered by them. There is no evidence of the existence of informal payments in Mexico. Contemporaneous household surveys indicated that those with fewer resources used a greater proportion of their income to pay for health events, and were even so high as to be considered catastrophic and/or "impoverishing" (Knaul & Frenk, 2005; Knaul et al., 2012). To measure the success of SPSS' implementation, indicators related to out-of-pocket health expenditure are continuously monitored.

Fifteen years after implementation, the expansion of public spending reversed the proportion paid by private sources of total health expenditure (Table 3.1). Studies have shown that the introduction of Seguro Popular reduced out-of-pocket expenses (García Díaz & Sosa-Rubí, 2011; Wirtz et al., 2013). However, out-of-pocket remains the main source of health financing and constituted 41.3% of total health expenditure in 2015 (Table 3.1). Out-of-pocket spending may have also decreased as a result of the promotion of generic drug policies and the growing prominence of the pharmacy–physician model, which reduces the cost of medical care generally associated with the purchase of medicines. However, such effects have not been investigated.

The reasons for incurring out-of-pocket expenses are diverse, ranging from reducing the long waiting times in the public sector to avoiding paying deductibles in private insurance (see section 3.5). Additionally, public services do not always have the medicines or supplies needed for care. This has driven a growing but heterogeneous group of private health providers, ranging from independent clinics, hospitals, to consultation rooms adjacent to pharmacy offices (CAF) affiliated to large chains and foundations. The latter have emerged as a solution to the needs of the low-income population, such as those covered by SPSS (39.1% report using a CAF) and those without any health insurance (30%), although these providers are also widely used by the publicly insured (González Block et al., 2018b). Figure 3.8 presents the breakdown of households by expense according to their socioeconomic level as reported in the National Household Income and Expenditure Survey 2016. It must be noted that no social insurance institution requires out-of-pocket payments from beneficiaries.

The probability of incurring drug expenses with a medical consultation is high, regardless of the service provider (public or private). The amount spent, however, has reduced over time. In 2008, two thirds of out-of-pocket expenses went to pay for medicines, while in 2016 it fell to only 32% (Figure 3.8) (Wirtz et al., 2013).

FIG. 3.8 Magnitude and composition of annual household out-of-pocket expenses by socioeconomic level, 2016

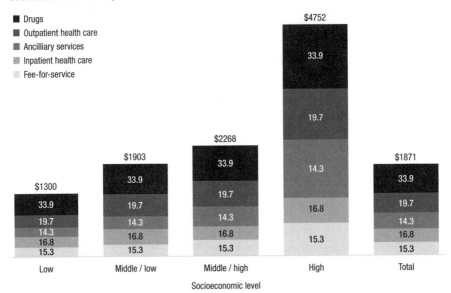

Note: Socioeconomic level established from the Mexican Association of Marketing Research and Public Opinion Agencies (AMAI) Classification

Source: INEGI (2016a)

3.5 **Voluntary health insurance**

3.5.1 *Role and size of the market*

As mentioned earlier, private health insurance covers 7.8% of the Mexican population (González Block et al., 2018b). Different products are offered in the market (personal accidents, major medical expenses, health care), with the product offering major medical expense coverage having the highest penetration. According to the Law on Insurance and Surety Institutions, indemnity insurance plans cover medical, hospital and other expenses to support the insured when they experience an accident or illness (Official Gazette of the Federation, 2003). These plans are offered in two categories: 1) individual, with unlimited coverage but high cost; and 2) group, with more limited coverage but lower cost premiums. The latter is designed for and mainly taken up by business groups and government. Collective, or group, insurance products constitute 73% of all health insurance products.

In 2015, private insurance generated 4.9% of total health expenditure and 10.6% of private spending on health in Mexico (Table 3.1). The share of total spending from private insurance has increased steadily over time, reaching a level 1.13 times higher in 2015 than the level in 2000 (2.3%). Similarly, as a proportion of total private spending, private insurance went from 4.2% in 2000 to 10.6% in 2015.

Private insurance is sought by the middle class as a means of complementing their social insurance; for which purpose insurance companies offer indemnity products through work-based collective enrolment, which offers relatively low levels of maximum indemnity coverage. These plans allow social insurance beneficiaries to avoid long wait times, access modern facilities and technology more quickly, and is possibly the only available way to access the most modern technology. Insurance companies also offer high-end plans through individual policies aimed at the relatively affluent self-employed. A recent study found that between 2007 and 2016, the number of privately insured grew by 66.7%, from 6.0 million to 9.9 million (González Block et al., 2018b).

3.5.2 *Market structure*

Private insurance is available without legal restrictions to individuals and firms wishing to purchase indemnity or health plans, although demand is concentrated in the middle socioeconomic strata. Population covered by private insurance is heterogeneous, as companies and governments buy it for their employees or organize the purchase of insurance by the beneficiaries themselves. The insurance market is highly concentrated: a total of 27 private insurance companies offer health insurance in the market, although only 10 offer insurance for major medical expenses. Furthermore, 76.8% of such policies are concentrated in five companies. Nationwide, nearly 40% of the policies were issued in the capital, Mexico City. Medical expenses are concentrated on hospitalizations costs (45%), medical fees (23%) and medications (18%). The diseases that concentrate the highest expenses are neoplasms, diseases of the digestive system, musculoskeletal system and connective tissue, as well as trauma and poisoning (González Block et al., 2018b).

■ **3.5.3** *Market behaviour*

Private insurance companies are regulated through the Law on Insurance and Surety Institutions (Diario Oficial de la Federación, 2013), and its operating instruments, such as the Insurance and Sureties Circular. This law stipulates how premiums are set, which starts from an actuarial calculation that considers individual health risks. In particular, insurance for illnesses and accidents includes frequency tables, average amounts, morbidity, loss ratio, as well as administrative expenses to be covered.

The benefits covered by insurers vary according to the type of policy. Indemnity insurance for medical expenses covers ambulatory, hospital and other services that are required for the recovery of the insured's health, as a consequence of an accident or illness. In this type of insurance, it is possible to find coverage of preventive care. Personal accident insurance covers the care of injuries or disability caused by an accident. In all cases, insurance reimburses health care expenditures post service utilization, based on prior agreements between the hospitals and the insurance agencies. In the case of health insurance policies sold through Special Health Insurance Institutions (ISES), preventive services are covered within a broad package of services free at the point-of-use.

The private insurance sector is poorly regulated, leading to the existence of market failures caused by an asymmetric relationship between patients, providers and insurers. When seeking care, the insured approach providers (medical specialists) who refer them to hospitals and guide them towards the services they require. It is common for physicians to receive economic incentives related to these referrals. According to studies, there is a concentration of demand in large hospitals located in large cities. Additionally, the treatments patients are guided towards choosing are not always consistent with clinical practice guidelines, which tends to raise the costs incurred by insurers. Insurers accept the prices dictated by the providers given the absence of homogeneous information systems for billing (González Block et al., 2018b).

■ **3.5.4** *Public policy*

Private medical insurance operates at the margins of public health policy, although efforts were made in the 1990s to integrate private health plans through linking ISES to health service purchasing by IMSS. However, this alternative lost political support soon after it was enacted, leading to the establishment of only a handful of ISES providers that cater to employees such as those in the banking industry who retained the right to self-manage their IMSS contributions. Furthermore, the López Obrador 2018–2024 administration eliminated public purchasing of indemnity insurance for high-ranking government employees. While IMSS is forbidden to sell services to any private purchaser, federal employees of the MoH are free to establish agreements with private insurance companies to bill for their services directly to insurers.

3.6 **Other sources of financing**

Although there are external sources of funding (donations, international agencies and civil society organizations), their contribution to health spending is minimal (less than 1%), according to the national expenditure accounts.

3.7 **Payment mechanisms**

The ways in which payments for services are made in the Mexican health system are heterogeneous and depend on the relationships between buyers and service providers (Table 3.4).

TABLE 3.4 Provider payment mechanisms

PROVIDERS	PAYERS				
	FEDERAL AND STATE GOVERNMENTS	SPSS	SOCIAL INSURANCE	PRIVATE INSURANCE	OUT-OF-POCKET
Outpatient service providers	Salary	Performance-based agreements, capitation	Salary	Fee-for-service (FFS)	
Hospitals	Budget	FFS	Budget	FFS, DRG, per diem	Per diem
Pharmacies	Wholesale purchasing through consolidated bids			Retail purchasing	
Public health services	Budget	Capitation	Budget	—	—

DRG: Payment by Diagnostic Related Groups; FSS: equivalent to the payment for service

Source: Authors

The federal and state governments and social insurance institutions, as purchasers, pay ambulatory service providers, hospitals and public health services through historical budgets. In the case of medicines, the purchase is consolidated among the different purchasers to increase competition among suppliers and reduce the possibility of high costs due to geographical differences.

SPSS introduced capitated payment for ambulatory and general hospital care and fee-for-service (FFS) for high-cost interventions paid through FPGC. Capitated payments were made from the federal CNPSS to the state-based financial administrators (REPSS), who allocated funds mostly to purchase inputs such as medicines or to hire additional medical personnel, or in some cases provide monetary supplements directly to providers. In some cases, FFS was also used to pay private providers for bundled packages of services such as laparoscopic surgery equipment and consumables. The provision of SPSS services was implemented in one state – Hidalgo – through hiring a private provider of primary care on a capitated basis. This modality was evaluated as cost-effective compared with the usual providers with respect to quality of care and the care of people with diabetes (Figueroa Lara, González Block & Alarcón Irigoyen, 2016).

It is worth mentioning that in order to make expenditure more efficient and to avoid the discretionary use of resources by state health payers, limits were applied to SPSS spending and to the consequent purchase of services. Only 40% of the amount transferred from the federal government to the states was able to be used to pay personnel, up to 30% to buy medicines covered by the FPGB, a minimum of 20% for health promotion, prevention and detection of diseases, and up to 6% to pay administrative and operating costs.

Finally, social insurance institutions and private insurance companies have made unsuccessful attempts to introduce hospital payment systems based on Diagnostic Related Groups, as a means of ensuring greater cost control. Cost control is a growing concern among private insurers, as studies suggest that the concentration of advanced technology in a limited number of private hospitals is leading to the inflation of hospital prices (González Block et al., 2018b).

4

Physical and human resources

■ Chapter summary

- Mexico's health system is characterized by an extensive yet ageing physical infrastructure now being complemented through diverse forms of public–private services agreements.
- Physical infrastructure is segmented within the public sector and between the public and private sectors, although service exchange agreements have tended to increase the efficiency of high-specialty services across public institutions.
- The private sector is growing mostly through investments in advanced technology, which supplement shortfalls in the public sector.
- Health information systems are playing an important role to improve public sector integration, although they have been unevenly developed across institutions.
- Human resources are regulated by national councils, with mandatory re-accreditation only for medical specialties.
- There are shortages of human resources, particularly of nurses and specialist physicians, while all health resources have a marked geographical imbalance favouring urban areas.

4.1 **Physical resources**

4.1.1 *Capital stock and investments*

Hospital investments and operational costs are highly integrated vertically within each social insurance institution, the MoH and state authorities. Private sector investments, for their part, are fully funded by private capital. Each public institution sets its own requirements according to its growth plans, leading often to overlapping infrastructure.

IMSS was originally planned to rely on private investment through the purchasing of private hospital services so an investment fund was not included in its financial architecture. However, it was decided in its first years of operation to establish an investment fund sourced from contributions that exclude the private sector and rely solely on its own resources and infrastructure. Today that fund has been depleted and IMSS relies on current contributions to plan investments, as well as on donations of plots of public land from local authorities. Notably, the first five hospitals in Mexico City were built with general fiscal contributions.

Financial and logistic constraints have resulted in governments and public agencies adding to hospital infrastructure through public–private services agreements (PPS). Governments and their agencies have also contracted out more expensive personal care services and the purchasing of "integrated health services", whereby consumables and capital equipment are paid for on the basis of cases treated. The MoH hospital network built the first PPS hospital in 2005 and now operates seven hospitals through this investment modality, while in 2018 IMSS and ISSSTE were in the process of building nine hospitals through PPS. Seguro Popular enabled the establishment of an investment fund leading to the construction of six high-specialty regional reference hospitals (HRAE), four of which were financed through PPS, as well as annexes to the National Cancer Institute. State authorities also invest in their own infrastructure, mostly through fiscal resources but the State of Mexico was able to finance two general hospitals through PPS (Astorga et al., 2016). Private sector investment is being stimulated through the purchasing of integrated health services, defined as the packaging of equipment, consumables and technical support to enable the in-house provision of specific services such as surgery, haemodialysis and imaging. Contracting-out is also increasing, although at a slow pace, to furnish services such as haemodialysis.

Private investment in health infrastructure is highly segmented, with a few groups participating in the building and equipping of hospitals of 50 beds or more, and small investors led by owner-physicians investing in small facilities. Private investment is now concentrating in high-technology diagnostic centres within and outside hospitals.

Health care investment is low, has decreased as a proportion of GDP and lags behind OECD standards (see section 3.1). Capital investment in health was 0.11% of GDP between 2003 and 2016, yet from 2013 this figure decreased to 0.08% for 2016. Average health investment for OECD countries is four times higher, or 0.39% of GDP over the same broader period (OECD, 2018a).

The regulation of capital investment is limited to the public sector and, within it, to investments in physical infrastructure by MoH and state authorities funded through MoH resources. The MoH provides certificates of need according to the Master Plan for Physical Infrastructure for Health (PMI), the infrastructure planning instrument managed by the General Directorate for Health Planning and Development (DGPLADES) whereby geographical accessibility is evaluated for specific types of medical infrastructure ranging from health centres to tertiary care hospitals (see sections 2.2.1 and 2.2.2). The rational utilization of high-specialty equipment and infrastructure is regulated across the public sector through agreements at the state level to exchange services according to a listing of agreed tariffs and a national mechanism to facilitate exchange and payment operated by DGPLADES.

■ **4.1.2** *Infrastructure*

PRIMARY CARE

There are 34 703 public and private health facilities registered in Mexico, of which 28 021 (80.7%) are outpatient clinics that provide primary care. Of the total number of primary care clinics, 21 286 (76%) are publicly owned and operated; of these, 14 332 (67.3%) belong to MoH. The IMSS-Bienestar also represents a large number of clinics with 4247 (20%), followed by IMSS with 1126 (5.2%) and ISSSTE with 1038 (4.8%). The remaining clinics are operated by federal, state, municipal and other health sector institutions such as SEDENA, SEMAR and PEMEX.

Up to 46.7% (9931) of the primary care clinics in the public sector correspond to fixed establishments located in rural areas and 41% (8736) are located in urban areas. The rest are represented by itinerant services, among which are Fortalecimiento de la Atención Médica Program (formerly Mobile Medical Units) and mobile brigades. These types of units aim to bring health services closer to people who live in communities whose geographical location is difficult to access.

According to the Report of the Observatory of Primary Care Services, in 2012 only 1.1% of primary care units had a clinical laboratory service and 0.5% had imaging services, mostly in urban areas (DGIS, 2018a). Of the total primary care clinics, 24% (6735) are privately owned and funded by the private medical sector, of which 86.7% are consulting rooms adjacent to pharmacies (DGIS, 2018a). Other sources have reported that there are about 60 000 private medical offices in Mexico, in which 67 855 doctors work as independent professionals, that offer, for the most part, the services of a single professional in solo practice (González Block et al., 2018b). The difference between the actual and registered number of units is explained by the fact that consulting rooms are usually not registered in the MoH's infrastructure catalogue, although they are accredited by COFEPRIS. According to the ENSANUT 2012 report, 39% of people who used outpatient health services did so in private units, which means that private care is an important entry point to the health system (Gutiérrez et al., 2012).

HOSPITAL UNITS

Mexico has a total of 4341 hospitals, of which 30% (1381) correspond to the public sector and are generally larger than private hospitals, which total 2960 (68%) (Table 4.1). Out of all public sector hospitals, 61% cater to the non-insured and 39% for the insured. Hospitals are distributed mostly in urban areas, while only 46 hospitals (3.3%) are located in rural areas (DGIS, 2018a).

Private sector hospitals totalled 3039 for 2003 and 2960 for 2015, a reduction mostly at the expense of smaller hospitals that went out of business partly as a result of the strengthening of MoH units since 2003 (Table 4.1). The vast majority of private hospitals (96%) are under 50 beds and up to 26% are very small units of one to four beds. Only 91 hospitals with 50 or more beds were in operation in 2013 and 94 in 2015, yet in this latter year they account for 62% of private sector hospital spending and 25% of discharges.

TABLE 4.1 Hospital units in the Mexican health system by institution, 2003 and 2015/2018

	2003[A, B]	%	2018[C, D]	%	YEARLY GROWTH, %
Hospitals	**4150**	**100**	**4341**	**100**	**0.3**
public sector	1111	27	1381	30	**1.6**
non-insured	536	48	838	61	**3.8**
MoH	462	86	751	90	**4.2**
IMSS-bienestar	69	13	80	10	**1.1**
University hospitals	5	1	7	1	**2.7**
Social insurance	**575**	**52**	**543**	**39**	**−0.4**
IMSS	349	61	268	49	**−1.5**
ISSSTE	106	18	111	20	**0.3**
PEMEX	23	4	23	4	**0.0**
SEDENA	42	7	45	8	**0.5**
SEMAR	34	6	33	6	**−0.2**
State and municipal governments	21	4	63	12	**13.3**
Private sector units by no. of beds	**3039**	**73**	**2960**	**68**	**−0.2**
1–4 beds	794	26	780	26	**−0.1**
5–9 beds	1309	43	1203	41	**−0.5**
10–14 beds	469	15	454	15	**−0.2**
15–24 beds	255	8	280	9	**0.7**
25–49 beds	137	5	149	5	**0.6**
50+ beds	75	2	94	3	**1.7**

Sources: [a]Public units: DGIS (2003), [b]Private units: INEGI. Información Estadística de Salud en Establecimientos Particulares, 2004, [c]Data for public units is for 2018 (DGIS, 2018b), [d]Data for private units is for 2015, cited in González Block et al. (2018b)

Up to 48% of the larger private hospitals with more than 50 beds are concentrated in Mexico City, Nuevo León and Jalisco, the three states with the largest urban concentrations. Private hospitals are mostly distributed in highly developed municipalities, with at least 95% of smaller hospitals between one and 24 beds located in municipalities classified as highly development according to the Human Development Index (González Block et al., 2018a).

HOSPITAL BEDS

With regard to hospital beds, a total of 123 465 were registered for 2018 in both the public and the private sectors (Table 4.2), giving a density of 1.0 beds per 1000 inhabitants. The public sector operates 76% of beds, with federal and state ministries of health having the largest number of beds, with 39 807, while IMSS has 33 361. Between 2013 and 2018, total beds increased by only 0.6%, which is not sufficient to keep up with population growth (see below).

TABLE 4.2 Hospital beds in the Mexican health system by institution and year, 2003 and 2015/2018

	2003[A]	%	2018[B, C]	%	YEARLY GROWTH, %
Beds	109 130	100	123 465	100	0.6
Public sector	75 974	70	89 485	76	1.2
Non-insured	34 077	45	42 797	48	1.7
MoH	31 549	93	39 807	93	1.7
IMSS-Bienestar	2181	6	2035	5	−0.4
University hospitals	347	1	955	2	11.7
Social insurance	41 897	55	46 688	52	0.8
IMSS	29 131	70	33 361	71	1.0
ISSSTE	6744	16	6861	15	0.1
PEMEX	985	2	922	2	−0.4
SEDENA	2527	6	2253	5	−0.7
SEMAR	1080	3	713	2	−2.3
State governments	1430	3	2578	6	5.4
Private sector	33 156	30	33 980	29	0.2

Sources: [a]DGIS (2015a), [b]Data for public beds is for 2018 (DGIS, 2018a), [c]Data for private beds is for 2015, cited in González Block et al. (2018b)

TABLE 4.3 Public sector hospital beds per 100 000 inhabitants at state level, 2000, 2010 and 2014

STATE	2000	2010	2014	% CHANGE 2000/2014
National average	**77.5**	**75.3**	**74**	**(4.5)**
Mexico City	189.2	175.6	177	(6.4)
Campeche	93.7	121.1	105	12.1
Sonora	104.8	100.9	100.3	(4.3)
Durango	80.2	90	97.3	21.3
Baja California Sur	142	82.3	91.5	(35.6)
Coahuila de Zaragoza	102.1	96.5	91.2	(10.7)
San Luis Potosí	56.7	63.5	88.6	56.3
Tamaulipas	96.7	86.2	87.1	(9.9)
Yucatán	89.2	76.3	84.7	(5.0)
Nuevo León	94.8	84.6	83.2	(12.2)
Jalisco	93.6	81.1	82.1	(12.3)
Colima	98.3	88.8	79.2	(19.4)
Chihuahua	76.7	75.7	76.2	(0.7)
Sinaloa	75.9	77.6	74.6	(1.7)
Tabasco	72.1	72.4	67.4	(6.5)
Aguascalientes	80.8	74	67.2	(16.8)
Puebla	65.5	61.2	65.2	(0.5)
Baja California	64.3	61.1	63.9	(0.6)
Zacatecas	49.2	62.7	63.9	29.9
Veracruz de Ignacio de la Llave	59.4	61.2	63.7	7.2
Nayarit	72.2	61.6	60.9	(15.7)
Quintana Roo	64.3	59.1	59.5	(7.5)
Morelos	53.1	52.2	56	5.5
Oaxaca	47.1	49.2	55.3	17.4
Guanajuato	50.7	53.4	55.2	8.9
Michoacán de Ocampo	46.6	54.1	55.1	18.2
Tlaxcala	50.1	55.5	54	7.8
Guerrero	50.6	49.5	52.6	4.0
México	53.1	47.6	49.3	(7.2)
Hidalgo	54.5	50.5	47.4	(13.0)
Querétaro	54	45.6	43.7	(19.1)
Chiapas	45.1	45.4	43.2	(4.2)

Source: INEGI (2016b)

Total public hospital beds are unevenly distributed across the country, with Mexico City being a clear outlier with 177 beds per 100 000 inhabitants as against the national average of 74 (Table 4.3). This situation is explained by the concentration of private large hospitals and of public High Specialty Hospitals in Mexico's largest city (Secretaría de Salud, 2016b). However, hospital bed densities are uneven across the rest of Mexican states, with Campeche having 105 beds per 100 000 inhabitants compared with Chiapas – one of Mexico's poorest states – with only 43.2. Bed density actually decreased by 4.5% at the national level between 2000 and 2014. Mexico City also showed a greater decrease, with states such as Baja California Sur reporting a decrease as high as 35.6%, and states such as San Luis Potosí an increase of 56.3%. While some changes may be due to investments or closures, it is also likely that changes may be due to specific reporting errors.

With regard to beds in private sector hospitals, they increased 0.2% per year from 2003 to 2013, a rate about a sixth that of the public sector (Table 4.2). Larger private hospitals have a very different services profile to their smaller counterparts, focusing more on diagnostic medicine and high-cost treatments requiring fewer beds (González Block et al., 2018b).

Mexico has the lowest density of hospital beds across OECD countries; the density of hospital beds in Mexico is lower than the density in Brazil (Table 4.4). The OECD average is 4.9 beds per 1000 inhabitants (including acute care, day care and others) and, according to OECD statistics, Mexico had 1.52 in 2016 – one third of the average density.

Mexico also has low levels of advanced technological equipment density with respect to OECD countries (Table 4.5). This situation can be attributed to generally low hospital investment in the public sector, together with the concentration of advanced technology in a few private hospitals, with social insurance and MoH hospitals lagging behind in needed investments.

TABLE 4.4 Hospital beds in acute hospitals per 1000 population in Mexico, OECD countries and Brazil, 2000, 2010 and 2016[a]

COUNTRY	2000	2010	2016
Mexico	**1.77**	**1.59**	**1.52**
Australia	4.04	3.78	—
Austria	7.95	7.65	7.42
Belgium	6.71	6.14	5.69
Canada	3.77	2.78	2.58
Chile	2.71	2.04	2.12
Czechia	7.8	7.04	6.85
Denmark	4.29	3.5	2.6
Estonia	7.04	5.27	4.76
Finland	7.54	5.85	3.97
France	7.97	6.43	6.05
Germany	9.12	8.25	8.06
Greece	4.77	4.48	4.2
Hungary	8.16	7.18	7
Iceland	—	3.58	3.13
Ireland	6.13	2.73	—
Israel	3.79	3.16	2.99
Italy	4.71	3.64	—
Japan	14.69	13.51	13.11

COUNTRY	2000	2010	2016
Korea	4.65	8.74	11.98
Latvia	8.77	5.68	5.72
Lithuania	8.83	7.16	6.69
Luxembourg	—	5.37	4.78
Netherlands	4.83	—	3.63
New Zealand	—	2.75	2.73
Norway	3.8	4.3	3.69
Poland	—	6.61	6.64
Portugal	3.71	3.37	3.42
Slovak Republic	7.86	6.46	5.78
Slovenia	5.4	4.57	4.49
Spain	3.65	3.12	2.97
Sweden	3.58	2.73	2.34
Switzerland	6.29	4.97	4.55
Turkey	2.05	2.52	2.75
United Kingdom	4.08	2.93	2.58
United States	3.49	3.05	—
Brazil (Non-OECD Economy)	2.82	2.36	—
OECD Average	5.75	4.94	4.90

[a]Includes day surgery and non-acute care beds

Source: OECD (2018c)

TABLE 4.5 CT and MRI equipment per million inhabitants in Mexico, compared with other countries in Latin America and OECD average, 2016

	TECHNOLOGY	COUNTRY/ REGION				
		MEXICO	BRAZIL[A]	CHILE[B]	COLOMBIA	OECD AVERAGE
CTS	Density	6.1	15.3	24.3	1.2	24.6
	Mexico vs others %	—	33.3	25.2	514	24.8
MRI	Density	2.6	6.8	12.3	0.2	15.6
	Mexico vs others %	—	32.0	20.9	1117	16.5
PET	Density	0.06	na	0.56	na	1.9
	Mexico vs others %	—	—	12.5	—	3.2
Gamma cameras	Density	0.40	1.6	1.6	na	7.9
	Mexico vs others %	—	24.5	29.4	—	5.1
Mammo-graphs	Density	9.5	na	14.8	na	22.4
	Mexico vs others %	—	—	64.2	—	42.5
Radiation therapy equipment	Density	1.6	na	2.3	na	7.5
	Mexico vs others %	—	—	58.3	—	21.7

na: not available

[a]Data for Brazil for 2012, compared with Mexico for same year. [b]Data for Chile for CTS and MR is for 2017, compared with Mexico for 2016

Note: Data is for 2014 and is compared with Mexico for same year unless stated otherwise

Source: OECD (2018c)

▪ 4.1.3 *Information technology and e-Health*

INFORMATION TECHNOLOGY

Information technology (IT) for health has been supported in Mexico mainly by IMSS through electronic medical records, the private sector through apps, and MoH hospitals and state-level health services through telehealth. While public efforts still fall short of using information technology to empower patients, a survey undertaken by PricewaterhouseCoopers' (PwC) Health Research Institute in Mexico suggested that close to a quarter of urban residents use information technology for health at least once a month (Health Research Institute, 2017). There is therefore great potential to reach out to patients through innovative information systems.

Use of electronic health records (ECE) is uneven and IMSS has made the greatest progress, with separate systems covering all their primary care and hospital facilities (González & López Santibañez, 2011). The MoH has ECE coverage in about 25% of its public hospitals and a handful of primary care systems, most notably in Querétaro where all primary care and hospital units are interconnected. The MoH regulates ECE development through an official norm to ensure that information can be transferred across hospitals and institutions. While Seguro Popular funded ECE projects prior to the 2009 crisis, since then a marked slowdown in new projects has been apparent, although gradual progress continues.

The MoH has focused its information technology efforts on developing telehealth capacity used for professional training and clinical and administrative support in community and specialty hospitals catering to the rural poor. Some form of telehealth capacity has been reported in 671 public sector medical units, of which 450 are within MoH hospitals. A recent study found that some 45 000 consultations were provided at MoH facilities in 15 states, supporting mostly mental health and internal medicine. In the highly rural state of Oaxaca, a total of 19 telehealth-equipped peripheral units and one central hospital offered 53 teleconferences and nearly 5000 consultations across five specialties, with maternal health a priority (Health Research Institute, 2017).

As noted above, MoH is concentrating on implementing the National Basic Health Information System (SINBA). Some information technology applications are being developed through this system, such as Radar CI-Salud, an app to help patients find over 28 000 public and private health provider units nationwide. IMSS is focused on making the most of its existing digital infrastructure, improving employer registration and developing a digital medical prescription system. It also developed and is now piloting an app to support early diabetes detection in high-risk individuals.

Within the private sector, IT is being developed to enable new care models closer to consumers through wellness and chronic disease management programmes, often supported by large firms. Models such as those implemented by Previta use mobile phones, the Internet and apps for managing chronic diseases (Health Research Institute, 2017). The Carlos Slim Foundation (FCS) has contributed to SINBA's consolidation of diabetes and hypertension reporting. FCS has also developed MIDO-Mi Salud, an app for chronic disease prevention, detection and care. The Inter-American Development Bank funded a pilot programme to improve patient adherence to diabetic treatments and lifestyle recommendations through cell phone messaging tailored to each population group's specific cultural context. Along the same lines, FCS is developing Apprende, a free access, cartoon-based app focused on patient education. FCS efforts are also now attempting to bring information technology into all MoH primary care units, focused on early pre-diabetes, diabetes and hypertension detection.

According to PwC, Mexico's audit and consulting firm, health apps are supporting service quality, equity and efficiency of the health system, while digital technology policy has increasingly been developed in the context of these wider system transformations (Health Research Institute, 2017). Telemedicine is growing in scale and scope, which improves service delivery and increases access to specialized medical care. IMSS' digital medicine prescription platform and diabetes detection app represent progress toward improving quality and efficiency. Technology is also enabling greater integration across public health institutions through online databases to support service exchange agreements (see section 6.5).

4.2 Human resources

4.2.1 Planning and registration of human resources

Health professionals are registered by the Ministry of Education based on Article 5 of the Constitution and its Statutory Law. Professionals obtain their professional license upon graduation from registered schools and universities and this is valid for life. Professional colleges can be freely formed by licensed individuals and each state government can recognize up to five colleges within any field of practice, coordinated by one national council or college. College membership is not obligatory, and no information is available regarding memberships with colleges in the health professions. However, the National College of Physicians (CMM) operating also as the National

Federation of Colleges of Medicine (FENACOME) has a membership of under 15 000, about 22% of all physicians in private practice. With the exception of medical specialists, no health care professional is required to recertify.

Medical specialists are regulated and governed through the Committee for Medical Specialty Councils (CONACEM), a body under the National Academy of Medicine (ANM), a non-profit, government-recognized and supported membership institution which has existed for over 150 years. CONACEM is mandated by the General Health Law to recognize and regulate 20 existing autonomous specialty councils. Councils are responsible only for certificate examinations, with training being the responsibility of medical colleges and associations. While the General Health Law was reformed in 2011 to mandate the recertification of specialists every 5 years, only close to 63% had been certified for 2016 (Saludiario, 2016). COFEPRIS is the authority in charge of enforcing certification, although this regulatory body has no oversight over IMSS physicians and does not prioritize the requirement. Public institutions tend not to require certification unless the hospital is participating in a certification process, as happens mostly with high specialty MoH hospitals seeking funding from FPGC. In the private sector, certification is driven by private hospitals as a requirement for clinical practice privileges.

Human resources planning is the joint responsibility of the MoH and the Ministry of Education (SEP). MoH and SEP coordinate the Interinstitutional Commission for the Training of Human Resources for Health (CIFRHS) with the participation of representatives from the Ministry of the Treasury and Public Credit, IMSS, ISSSTE, the National System for Integral Family Development (DIF), the National Council of Technical Professional Education (CONALEP), the National Association of Universities and Institutions of Higher Education (ANUIES), the ANM and the CINSHAE. Among CIFRHS' chief tasks is the management of the National System of Medical Residencies whereby residents are selected and agreements recognized between schools and faculties of medicine, specialty councils and training hospitals. Training hospitals are mostly in the public sector, with only a handful of medical schools having their own teaching hospitals and only a few of the largest private hospitals participating in medical training.

The National System of Medical Residencies selects residency candidates through the National Exam for Medical Residency Candidates (ENARM). In 2017, a total of 8780 residents were admitted for 26 specialty areas in 46 faculties or schools, mostly determined by the number of training opportunities rather than the demand or need for specialists by public and private institutions (CIFRHS, 2017). These considerations are the remit of CIFRHS' Committee for the Study of Human Resources in Health Training Needs, which ultimately depend on human resource contracting decisions taken independently and with little coordination by the multitude of public and private health provision institutions.

■ **4.2.2** *Health workforce trends*

There is no unified source for workforce statistics in Mexico. Public sector institutions report directly to the MoH, while private sector data is only available for hospitals through annual census surveys undertaken by INEGI. Private sector personnel outside hospitals are estimated through annual National Occupation and Employment Surveys (ENOE) also undertaken by INEGI. Important differences exist between ENOE data for public health sector employees and data directly reported by institutions to MoH. While some of these differences can be attributed to sampling error, it is also likely that institutional information is imprecise, particularly for some categories such as medical specialists.

It is worth noting at the outset that the distribution of physician employment has favoured the public sector relative to the private sector. In 2000, about 59% of physicians were employed in the public sector, while by 2016 it had increased to 71% (González Block et al., 2018b). This is partly due to the relative growth of the public sector, together with better remuneration of those employed by the government in comparison to privately employed generalist physicians. Also noteworthy, salary differences between Mexican physicians and those in OECD countries are large, with average yearly earnings for generalists being US$ 44 040 PPP in Mexico compared with US$ 78 039 in the OECD, and for specialists US$ 58 451 in Mexico compared with US$ 109 282 in the OECD (2018c).

It is also important to note the limitations of human resource density statistics offered by the MoH (and hence by the OECD), and the discrepancies this information has with respect to ENOE data. The MoH reports human resources data based on two sources: open contract information provided by public institutions and an annual census of private hospitals. Open contract information leads to double counting, particularly of specialized physicians, given that a significant number of them work for several public institutions as well as across the public and private sectors. On the other hand, the census misses human resources personnel employed outside hospitals or who practise in hospitals but are paid directly by patients or insurers. Given these limitations, the most reliable source of information regarding human resources in health is ENOE, on account of its considering a sample of people employed in the health economy which avoids double counting or underreporting. Furthermore, ENOE uses a similar classification of professions as the MoH and OECD, thus providing consistency across specialized and non-specialized resources. Therefore, ENOE information is used to describe general human resource density, noting any relevant discrepancies with MoH and OECD data.

When considering all practising physicians, in 2016 there were 1.9 physicians per 1000 inhabitants according to ENOE, compared with the OECD average of 3.3 (Table 4.6). It is worth noting that double counting – in spite of underreporting human resources in the private sector – leads the OECD to report for Mexico a total of 2.4 physicians per 1000 inhabitants.

TABLE 4.6 Health workforce for selected categories according to information source, sector of employment and density, 2016

	INFORMATION SOURCE						
	OECD[A]			ENOE (MEXICO)[B]			
	MEXICO		OECD COUNTRIES RATE PER 1000	PUBLIC	PRIVATE	TOTAL	RATE PER 1000
	TOTAL	RATE PER 1000					
Total physicians	286 685	2.4	3.3	163 067	67 855	230 922	1.9
General and family medicine	106 108	0.9	1.0	107 708	52 192	159 900	1.3
Specialists	180 577	1.5	2.2	55 359	15 663	71 022	0.6
Dentists	16 798	0.1	0.7	19 748	78 254	98 002	0.8
Total nurses	350 953	2.9	8.9	314 853	27 397	342 250	2.8
Specialists	208 479	1.7	7.2	186 726	11 266	197 992	1.6
Technical	142 474	1.2	1.7	128 127	16 131	144 258	1.2

Note: Information is based on working-age population sample data at the national level

Sources: [a]OECD (2018c), [b]INEGI (2016)

GENERAL PHYSICIANS

The total physician workforce in Mexico according to ENOE was of 230 922, of whom 163 067 (71%) declared either the federal or state governments as their primary employer (Table 4.6). Among general physicians, 11% of those within the public sector report a second employment, while 14% employed in the private sector report likewise. Mexico has a lower density of general physicians than the OECD average, at 0.9 compared with 1.0 per 1000 inhabitants.

The distribution of general physicians across states is uneven. Among physicians employed in the public sector and private hospitals and using official MoH data, the lowest density is 0.6 per 1000 inhabitants for the State of Mexico, increasing to 1.2 for the state of Campeche (Figure 4.1). Mexico City is an outlier, with a density of close to 1.8. A greater concentration in richer states such as Mexico City, Jalisco and Nuevo León would be expected for physicians in private employment outside hospitals, for whom data is not available. Concentration of physicians in urban areas has been a historical problem due to fewer opportunities for professional and family development in rural areas.

FIG. 4.1 General physicians per 10 000 inhabitants by state, 2005 and 2014

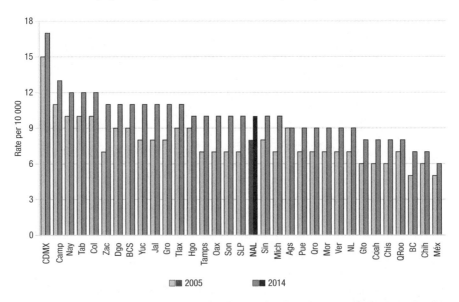

Ags: Aguascalientes; BC: Baja California; BCS: Baja California Sur; Camp: Campeche; CDMX: Mexico City; Chis: Chiapas; Chih: Chihuahua; Coah: Coahuila; Col: Colima; Dgo: Durango; Gro: Guerrero; Gto: Guanajuato; Hgo: Hidalgo; Jal: Jalisco; Mex: Estado de México.; Mich: Michoacán; Mor: Morelos; NAL: National average; Nay: Nayarit; NL: Nuevo León; Oax: Oaxaca; Pue: Puebla; Qro: Querétaro; QRoo: Quintana Roo; Sin: Sinaloa; SLP: San Luis Potosí; Son: Sonora; Tab: Tabasco; Tamps: Tamaulipas; Tlax: Tlaxcala; Ver: Veracruz; Yuc: Yucatán; Zac: Zacatecas

Source: Secretaría de Salud (2016b)

General physicians increased in number in public employment and in private hospitals by 26% between 2005 and 2014 (not reported for solo-practising private physicians; Secretaría de Salud, 2016b). Increases were especially notable within public MoH hospitals due to a boost in employment following Seguro Popular implementation (Figure 4.2).

FIG. 4.2 General physicians in Mexico, 2005–2014

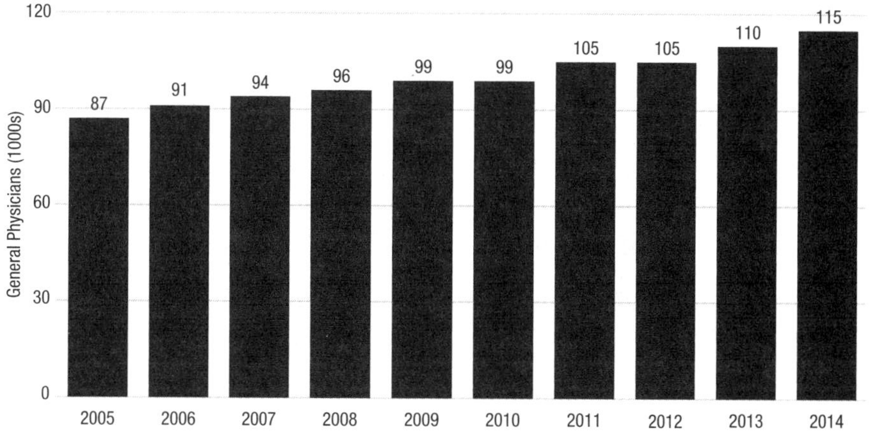

Source: Secretaría de Salud (2016b)

MEDICAL SPECIALISTS

According to ENOE reporting, medical specialists in both the public and private sectors totalled 71 022 for 2016. This figure is considerably lower than the 180 577 reported to the MoH and OECD by institutions and private hospitals. This discrepancy is most likely due to double counting of open contracts, in spite of the exclusion of private sector specialists working outside hospitals.

With respect to ENOE data, a total of 55 359 (61%) specialists are employed in the public sector and the remaining 15 663 (39%) are employed by hospitals in the private sector. ENOE also reports that 33% of specialists in the public sector have more than one place of employment, and that for 12.7% the private sector is their primary employer (González Block et al., 2018b). Such double employment rates help explain the double counting identified in the OECD data.

Specialists are unevenly distributed across the country and, according to MoH data, density ranges between 2.5 and over 4 specialists per 1000 inhabitants in the cases of the states of Mexico City and Nuevo León, respectively, and as low as 0.4 per 1000 in the poor state of Chiapas (Figure 4.3). Numbers of medical specialists have increased at a slower rate than generalists; at a rate of 4% per annum between 2005 and 2014 (Figure 4.4) (Secretaría de Salud, 2016b, p. 54). The actual growth rates may be lower than reported here, as they are based on the sources of information that may be affected by double counting.

The gap between the supply and demand of medical specialists will increase given the current rate of licensing new graduates and retirement rates, together with the rising health care needs of a growing, ageing population (Fajardo Dolci, 2014). Considering just the public sector, it is estimated that in 2030 nearly 165 000 specialists will be required to maintain the current supply of 1.2 specialists per 1000 persons. However, given current trends, it is estimated that the actual number will be somewhere near 124 600, suggesting a deficit of some 40 400 specialists or 32.4% of the total. However, if an increase of 15% in demand is considered given population growth and ageing, the gap would be 47% of these expected numbers. Experts agree that it is reasonable to expect an increase of up to 30% of current demand, in which case the deficit would be 65% of current specialist supply (Santacruz Varela et al., 2015). Taking cardiology as an example, it is estimated that in 2030 a total of 463 additional specialists will be required considering population growth and current demand rates. The gap between available cardiologists and the demand for them will grow to a deficit of between 773 and 1082 professionals with increases in demand of between 15% and 30%, respectively.

DENTISTS

The total number of Mexican dentists was just over 98 000 according to ENOE data for 2016, of which 19 748 (20%) are employed in the public sector and the rest in the private sector. Dentist density according to ENOE is 0.8 per 1000 inhabitants, higher than the OECD average of 0.7. It is important to note that MoH, and hence OECD, density figures for dentists are much lower given they work mostly outside hospitals in the private sector.

FIG. 4.3 Distribution of medical specialists per 10 000 inhabitants, by state, 2005 and 2014

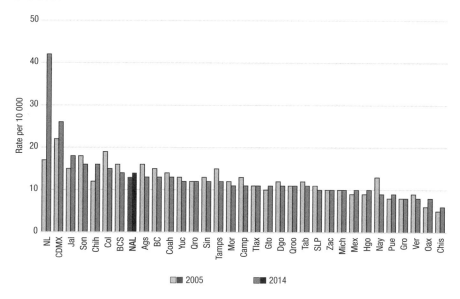

Ags: Aguascalientes; BC: Baja California; BCS: Baja California Sur; Camp: Campeche; CDMX: Mexico City; Chis: Chiapas; Chih: Chihuahua; Coah: Coahuila; Col: Colima; Dgo: Durango; Gro: Guerrero; Gto: Guanajuato; Hgo: Hidalgo; Jal: Jalisco; Mex: Estado de México.; Mich: Michoacán; Mor: Morelos; NAL: National average; Nay: Nayarit; NL: Nuevo León; Oax: Oaxaca; Pue: Puebla; Qro: Querétaro; QRoo: Quintana Roo; Sin: Sinaloa; SLP: San Luis Potosí; Son: Sonora; Tab: Tabasco; Tamps: Tamaulipas; Tlax: Tlaxcala; Ver: Veracruz; Yuc: Yucatán; Zac: Zacatecas.
Source: Secretaría de Salud (2016b)

FIG. 4.4 Specialized physicians, 2005–2014

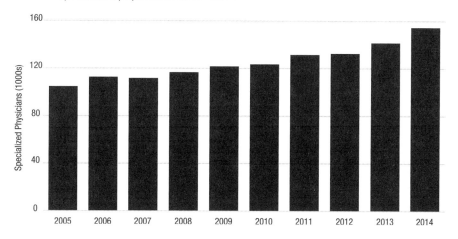

Source: Secretaría de Salud (2016b)

NURSES

The total number of nurses was just above 342 000 according to ENOE data. Nurses with a professional degree amount to just below 198 000, with the remainder being technical personnel with high school education. Nurse density is 2.8 per 1000 inhabitants, a figure that is a third lower than the OECD average of 7.2. It is interesting to note that hospital nurses in the public sector earn US$ 31 269 PPP, compared with the OECD average of US$ 47 599, a much smaller difference than with respect to physicians. Mexico has a relatively low density of both nurses and physicians compared with other OECD countries, with a similar rate for both, whereas in most OECD countries nurse density is higher than physician density (Figure 4.5).

FIG. 4.5 Practising nurses and physicians per 1000 population, 2016 or latest

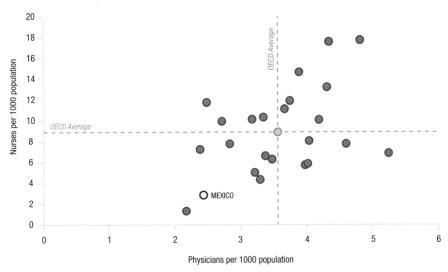

Source: OECD (2018c)

HEALTH ADMINISTRATORS

Neither the public nor private sectors require specialized administrators to fill the medical or operations director roles in Mexican hospitals. There are no official statistics enabling the identification of professional administrators within the health system; a few universities and postgraduate programmes offer specialized administration training (see below).

■ **4.2.3** *Professional mobility of health workers*

Health professionals in Mexico tend to be trained in country and are sourced mostly from Mexican nationals. Few health professionals emigrate to work in other countries, in spite of the high demand in the United States and Canada. However, no official or research-based information is available, and it may be that a significant number of nurses migrate to these North American countries.

■ **4.2.4** *Training of health workers*

Undergraduate training of health professionals totalled close to 60 000 graduates in 2017 across seven major health professions, with an annual growth rate of 7.8% since 2011, which is nearly seven times the general population growth (Table 4.7). A total of 155 undergraduate medical training programmes report to the Ministry of Education, of which 103 are registered by the Mexican Association of Faculties and Schools of Medicine (AMFEM) while 75 are accredited by the Mexican Council for Accreditation of Medical Education (COMAEM) (ANFEM, 2018). Programmes are distributed in all but one state, Baja California Sur (AMFEM, 2016; ANUIES, 2017). Over 13 000 physicians graduated in 2017, with a 2.3% per year increase since 2011, which is double the growth rate of the general population. The total number of programmes has more than doubled since 2011, when 77 were reported by the Ministry of Education. Yet since then, the number of medical graduates has only increased by 13.8%, suggesting that these new schools have thus far recruited only a small number of students. The growth rate of medical graduates was most notable in the first decade of the new century; while in 1998 a total of 64 medical training programmes graduated 5187 doctors, in 2011 the number of graduates doubled from about the same number of schools (Flores Echavarría et al., 2001).

In 2017, close to half of medical schools were private, although these are smaller in size than their public counterparts. Public schools are mostly dependent on federal and state budgets and provide free education, while private medical schools are supported through student fees and receive few if any government subsidies, except for training in public hospitals. Medical training programmes can be freely established by universities or other academic institutions, requiring only minimum standards to be guaranteed to federal regulators.

Health professions and authorities play a small role in determining student intake. AMFEM accredits faculties and schools following a rigorous, peer-supported system. Medical undergraduate programmes are concentrated in Mexico City, followed by Jalisco, Tamaulipas and Baja California, with between 7 and 12 units, which are largely or mostly private and cater to foreign students, mostly from the United States. A key issue with Mexican medical education is its focus on hospital and specialty care to the relative neglect of the development of training curricula oriented to primary care and health promotion and prevention, although numerous efforts have been made towards this end.

Nursing has traditionally been treated as a technical career, requiring only 9 years of basic education followed by full-time training for 3 years at a technical school. Nonetheless, undergraduate nursing training is among the fastest growing health profession, training over 14 000 nurses per year with an annual growth of 18.2% since 2011 (Table 4.7). Currently, this number is only slightly above the number of training medical professionals, although it will soon surpass it given the differences in growth rates between the two professions.

TABLE 4.7 Graduates in health sciences, 2011 and 2017

RESOURCE	2011	2017	% CHANGE	% ANNUAL GROWTH
Medicine	11 550	13 148	13.8	2.3
Nursing	6736	14 077	109.0	18.2
Odontology	5178	5302	2.4	0.4
Psychology	14 642	19 441	32.8	5.5
Nutrition	2017	5369	166.2	27.7
Pharmaceutical chemistry	518	1909	268.5	44.8
Other[a]	103	507	392.2	65.4
Total	**40 744**	**59 753**	**46.7**	**7.8**

[a]Includes health promotion, health education and health management, among others

Source: ANUIES (2017)

Dentists are trained in faculties in most cases separate from those of medicine and have shown stagnation in graduation numbers since 2011, with only 0.4% growth per year. Graduation of psychologists is the largest among the health professions, with over 19 000 per year and a yearly growth rate of 5.5%, which is partly explained by their strong demand in human resource departments within services and industry, less so by the demand within the health sector. Nutritionists are the third fastest growing profession, with 27.7% growth per year, partly explained by industry demand as well as within the health sector due to the overweight and obesity epidemics.

In Mexico, pharmacy and laboratory professionals are trained through a single pharmaceutical chemistry curriculum catering to the medical laboratory and the pharmacy sectors. This integration is partly explained by the limited demand for pharmacy specialists due to the country's permissive regulation of drug dispensation. However, training for these professionals has observed strong growth at 44.8% annual increase since 2011, although still too low to make a significant change to the safety and quality of drug dispensation.

Training of professionals in areas such as health promotion, education and management has increased the fastest across the health sciences, although starting from a very small base and still insufficient to alter Mexico's human resource needs. In 2011, 103 professionals graduated from these disciplines, compared with a 65.4% increase in 2017, which saw 507 students graduating from a total of 37 programmes.

SECONDARY PROFESSIONAL TRAINING (SPECIALIZATION)

Mexico graduates 12 medical specialists per 100 000 inhabitants, a larger number than the OECD average of 10. However, Mexico remains far below the density of medical specialists observed within the OECD (Fajardo Dolci, 2014). Notably, since 2011 there have been more female than male residents being accepted.

Demand for medical specialty training is high with respect to supply, with only 7805 new entrants accepted in 2016 out of 35 087 candidates (22%) (Ramiro et al., 2017). Intake to basic specialties such as internal medicine, paediatrics and gynaecology and obstetrics is lower, accepting only one out of every six to eight candidates. Acceptance to some other specialties is still lower, with only one out of 24 candidates accepted for ear, nose and throat, and 1 in 45 for radiation oncology.

Demand for specialty training has increased significantly since 2001, when 18 023 general physicians sought entry and 3362 were accepted. In 2016, these figures grew by 95% in demand and 132% in acceptances. While growth in enrolment has averaged 8.2% per year, much higher than population growth, it is still insufficient to cover for specialist retirement, which occurs at a very high rate especially within IMSS. Indeed, up to 15 000 IMSS specialists are expected to retire between 2014 and 2024 – about 1500 per year; most are below 60 years of age. Unsurprisingly, IMSS is among the health institutions with highest student intake, with an annual growth in residents of 19.6% between 2001 and 2016. Most residents graduate from the family medicine specialty and fill positions in primary care.

Accreditation and continuing education are only mandatory for medical specialists; they are not mandatory for general practitioners. Medical colleges and the National Academy of Medicine provide continuing education courses regulated by the Specialist Councils and the Council for General Medicine. There are no official statistics on the characteristics and performance of continuing education.

■ **4.2.5** *Career paths in the health professions*

Physician employment within hospitals and across the health system is little regulated and each institution follows its own procedures regarding career paths. In the public sector, appointments to the posts of service chief and hospital director are usually tied to trade union relations and political appointments. Within IMSS, directors of its 27 High Specialty Hospitals are appointed by employer, employee and government representatives sitting on hospital consulting councils. A study of the quality of consulting council decisions at these hospitals revealed that neither appointment criteria nor procedures are explicit, and councils appoint a new director for each hospital every 2.8 years, on average. Past directors return to operational positions as trade-unionized staff (González Block, 2018). In the private sector, the hospitals larger than 50 beds do not appoint medical specialists and employ only in-house physicians for emergency care and diagnostic services. Most physicians are self-employed and gain clinical practice privileges through approval by a hospital medical committee reporting to the owners. Smaller hospitals tend to be family businesses, with family members filling in specific appointments.

Public institutions organize training for professional and non-professional staff through joint trade union employer committees and through institutional bureaux. However, professional mobility is not tied to accreditation nor to compliance with specific training standards. Many training opportunities open to physicians in both the public and private sector are sponsored by the pharmaceutical industry, overseen by the ethics watchdog Council for Ethics and Transparency of the Pharmaceutical Industry (CETIFARMA) and through courses approved by colleges and councils.

5

Provision of services

■ Chapter summary

- The MoH conducts and regulates national public health policy through interinstitutional collaboration strategies.
- Primary care is delivered through independent provider networks for specific population groups.
- While governmental health institutions do not allow the choice of primary care physician, patients pay out-of-pocket to access physicians in pharmacies or clinics outside their insurer's provider network.
- Primary care teams operate as a gateway to specialized and hospital care within their own networks and provide a wide range of curative, prevention and health promotion services including vaccination, family planning, prenatal care and paediatric care.
- Specialized public ambulatory care is scarce: institutional provider networks include most services within proprietary facilities, distinguishing between general and specialized ambulatory care, general (second level) hospitalization and high-specialty (third level) hospitalization.
- While the Mexican pharmaceutical market is the second largest in Latin America, Mexico does not have an integrated pharmaceutical policy.

- A voluntary notification programme for adverse drug events operates across the health system, but lacks systematized reporting by health professionals.
- Drug dispensation is operated by each public provider network within their own facilities, free of charge.
- Rehabilitation for people with disabilities is provided by public and private non-profit institutions.
- Intermediate care aimed at reducing hospitalizations is offered by the MoH network through specialized ambulatory care centres.
- Permanent long-term care is only provided by the private sector for a limited segment of the population.
- Palliative care is only available in a few highly specialized public and private hospitals.
- Mental health care services are mostly concentrated in a few specialized hospitals, and ambulatory and community programmes are lacking.

5.1 Public health

The MoH regulates and largely finances disease prevention interventions through health promotion and education and the coordination of epidemiological surveillance systems (see sections 2.2.1 and 2.2.2). State health authorities are responsible for the coordination and implementation of public health initiatives, prompted mainly by MoH and social insurance providers. The MoH leads public health policy and strategy through the Undersecretary of Prevention and Health Promotion, which regulates the provision of public health programmes for geographically isolated populations through coordination across MoH, social insurance and private sector provider networks. The undersecretary also funds public health programmes benefiting the uninsured and, in some cases, whole populations regardless of insurance status.

- The General Directorate for Health Promotion (DGPS) establishes the policies and strategies to be followed for the development of health promotion initiatives that contribute to the improvement and conservation of Mexico's physical, mental and social health.

- The General Directorate of Reproductive Health (DGSR) designs and operates mechanisms to strengthen actions in the provision of maternal health services, newborn health, prevention and control of cervical and breast cancer, family planning and the sexual and reproductive health of teenagers.
- The National Epidemiological Surveillance Centre (SINAVE) coordinates the national policy on the prevention and control of communicable and noncommunicable diseases, responds to epidemiological emergencies and disasters, accidents, adult and elderly health, prevention and treatment of oral health, and manages epidemiological surveillance.
- The National Centre for the Health of Children and Adolescents (CENSIA) determines and evaluates compliance with national policies on the health of children and adolescents and vaccination policies for the entire population.
- The National Centre for the Prevention and Control of HIV/ AIDS (CENSIDA) develops policies and strategies on prevention, treatment and control of the human immunodeficiency virus infection, acquired immunodeficiency syndrome and transmission of sexual infections.

Two other federal bodies involved in the stewardship and execution of public health actions are: 1) the National Commission against Addictions (CONADIC), responsible for developing and implementing the national policy on addiction and mental health care; and 2) COFEPRIS, responsible for both designing and executing the national policy on medicines and other medical supplies, and the prevention and control of the harmful effects of environmental factors on human health, occupational health and basic sanitation (Secretaría de Gobernación, 2012).

IMSS executes public health actions through the Integrated Health Programmes (PrevenIMSS), a strategy to promote health, nutrition, prevention, detection and control of diseases, as well as reproductive health. PrevenIMSS focuses on programmatic age groups: children under 10, adolescents 10 to 19, women, men (both groups 20 to 59) and older adults (60 and older) (Muñoz, 2006). The ISSSTE operates the Preventive Care Model (PrevenISSSTE) that includes: 1) an online, interactive platform providing information and assessment of risk factors for chronic degenerative diseases, overweight and obesity, and substance abuse, and offering recommendations for healthy habits; 2) a call centre providing professional advice and guidance on health problems; and 3) the PrevenISSSTE modules in health clinics and hospitals that provide patient guidance based on the online health risk assessment platform and that refer patients for further tests and to their family physicians (PrevenISSSTE, 2020).

At the state level, the operation of public health programmes is the responsibility of the state health services and delegations of social insurance institutions and other public sector health institutions. These efforts cover both urban and rural areas and extend to sparsely populated rural areas and Indigenous communities. State health services operate through regional operation and coordination offices, referred to as Sanitary Jurisdictions, which are technical and administrative departments responsible for the operation of health programmes for a group of municipalities. Sanitary Jurisdiction offices do not provide health services of their own but include administrative and supervisory teams responsible for health centre logistics and for monitoring health programme activities and care processes at health centres in a specific area. While the structure of health jurisdictions varies, it generally comprises two branches: one dedicated to the operation of MoH primary care facilities for the uninsured, and another dedicated to the planning, operation and supervision of public health programmes for the entire population, usually in coordination with social insurance institutions and less so with private providers.

The scope of responsibilities under sanitary jurisdictions has gradually decreased, mostly as a result of moving sanitary risk protection and programme monitoring up to the state level and through the reduction in fee-for-service (FFS) charges with Seguro Popular implementation. A new role has been envisioned for sanitary jurisdictions to coordinate health care through the Comprehensive Health Care Model (MAIS), seeking to overcome rigidities in the segmented and fragmented care system, while prioritizing health promotion and disease prevention. Though not yet implemented, the MAIS was envisioned to create and regulate health care networks through priority health interventions in their demographic and epidemiological contexts, with the perspective of facilitating continuous and coordinated care. The MAIS faces diverse challenges for its implementation given the heterogeneous and segmented public and private institutions and providers (Secretaría de Salud, 2015b).

A few municipal governments also carry out health promotion programmes, such as the MoH-supported Healthy Environments and Communities Programme, which focuses on disease prevention and control. In most cases, however, such programmes are limited to the vaccination of dogs against rabies or the control of prostitution. Other public institutions, such as the social services agency the National System for Integral Family Development (DIF), provide social and health assistance to vulnerable population groups through public centres for the elderly and children.

The MoH has strengthened strategic public health programmes against tobacco use, addictions, overweight and obesity, and diabetes, and is responsible for programmes to increase the coverage of vaccination and neonatal screening. The MoH has also strengthened the Epidemiological Surveillance System and sectoral coordination for public health actions. These cases are described below.

5.1.1 *Regulation on the use of tobacco*

In 2008, the General Law for Tobacco Control was enacted, empowering the MoH to take health protection measures against risks associated with the consumption of tobacco products, including demand-reduction measures (Cámara de Senadores de los Estados Unidos Mexicanos, 2008). Regulations enacted in 2009 and 2012 introduced mandatory labelling of tobacco products while state-level legislation has sought to curb second-hand smoke (Secretaría de Salud, 2009a; Cámara de diputados, 2012; Rubio, Rubio Monteverde & Álvarez Cordero, 2011). Although the effectiveness of these and other measures have been questioned (Barrientos, 2010), the results of the National Survey of Addictions (ENA 2008; Consejo Nacional Contra las Adicciones et al., 2009) and the National Survey of Drug, Alcohol and Tobacco Consumption (ENCODAT) 2016–2017 (Reynales Shigamatsu et al., 2017) show a significant decrease in the prevalence of tobacco consumption in the Mexican population for those aged 12 to 65 (20.4% in 2008 to 17.6% in 2016). Similarly, the age of onset of daily consumption among Mexican smokers aged 12 to 65 years increased from 16.7 years in 2008 to 19.3 years in 2016.

■ **5.1.2** *Universal vaccination programme*

The Universal Vaccination Programme of Mexico enjoys international recognition, being public and free and among the most complete schemes worldwide, with coverage against 15 preventable diseases (Díaz Ortega et al., 2012). However, Mexico is an extremely complex country in its geography and in the capacity for sectoral and intersectoral coordination, limiting coverage in practice. According to the National Mid-Way Health and Nutrition Survey 2016, coverage of the complete vaccination scheme in children under 12 months was 51.7% (range: from 67.6% for the pentavalent vaccine (PV) to 93.9 %, for the Bacillus Calmette-Guerin (BCG) vaccine); in children 12–23 months, 53.9% (range: from 68.5% for the triple viral vaccine (SRP) to 98.3% for BCG), and 63.2% for children 24–35 months (range: from 85.3% for the pneumococcal vaccine to 98.6% for BCG). In children of 6 years of age, coverage of one dose of SRP was 97.8%, and for two doses, 50.7%. Among the main explanatory variables identified for coverage deficiencies was being the child of a mother speaking an Indigenous language. This indicates that both the monitoring of the scheme and the universality of the vaccination programme must be strengthened to reach all social strata, respecting their traditions and culture (INSP, 2012).

The survey also revealed that coverage at 1 year of age of BCG, hepatitis B and pentavalent vaccines was greater than 90.0%. However, important differences can be noted across states, ranging between 77.7% and 84.6%, as well as across vaccines, with coverage of pneumococcal vaccine being 87.6%, for rotavirus 76.8%, and 81.2% for the combined vaccine against measles, mumps and rubella (MMR). The national vaccination coverage of the full scheme at 1 year of age reached 60.7% and increased to 74.2% for the four-vaccine scheme; while in children up to 2 years old, these coverages were 64.5% and 77.9%, respectively. These last figures are well above those reported for 2000, of 26.5% and 50%, respectively.

■ **5.1.3** *Extended neonatal screening*

Neonatal screening is recognized as the second most effective preventive practice in the world, second only to vaccination. Neonatal screening is obligatory in all institutions that care for neonates according to the Official Mexican

Standard for Health Information for the care of women during pregnancy, childbirth and puerperium and the newborn (Diario Oficial de la Federación, 1988; Secretaría de Salud, 1995). Although only the detection of congenital hypothyroidism – basic screening – was declared mandatory, a new standard for the prevention and control of birth defects was decreed in 2014, mandating the expanded neonatal screening for the detection of inborn errors of metabolism (Diario Oficial de la Federación, 2014). With the new regulatory framework, a large number of institutions in Mexico are already conducting studies of expanded neonatal screening (Trigo Madrid et al., 2014).

■ 5.1.4 *National Strategy for the Prevention and Control of Overweight, Obesity and Diabetes*

The federal government responded to Mexcio's obesity and diabetes epidemics by launching the National Strategy for the Prevention and Control of Overweight, Obesity and Diabetes (ENCSOD) in 2013 and declaring diabetes mellitus (DM) a national epidemiological emergency in 2016. ENCSOD combines public health, medical care and fiscal and regulatory policies. The MoH established the Mexican Observatory of Non-Communicable Diseases and partnered with the FCS to develop a chronic disease information system known as MIDO. It includes mobile health tools, a patient-monitoring system and modules to monitor drug supplies and personnel training. MIDO has been installed in more than 12 000 MoH primary care centres nationwide, enabling monitoring of diabetes quality indicators. Monitoring resulted in an increase of HbA1c tests – the gold standard for diabetes control – to 48% of patients from 14% (Health Research Institute, 2017).

- As part of its strategy, MoH, in collaboration with the Ministry of Finance and Public Credit, decreed the Special Tax on Products and Services (IEPS) of 1 peso per litre for sugary drinks from 2014. This tax has placed Mexico at the forefront of international public health measures against chronic diseases. The revenues raised are used for the construction of school drinking fountains, strengthening the coverage of drinking-water services in rural locations, and for the promotion, prevention and disease programmes related to the fight against malnutrition, overweight and obesity. During the first 2 years of implementation, purchases of drinks with taxes were reduced by 8.5% per year on average, and those of water and other beverages without taxes increased by 2.1% (Colchero et al., 2017). However, overweight and obesity among adults still increased from 71.3%· in 2012 to 75.2% in 2018 (INEGI nd).

- When comparing the results of the ENSANUT 2012 and 2016 reports, the combined prevalence of overweight and obesity among 5- to 11-year-olds decreased from 34.4% in 2012 to 33.2% in 2016. In adolescents between 12 and 19 the prevalence of combined overweight and obesity was 36.3%, higher than in 2012 (34.9%). In adults 20 years of age and older, the combined prevalence of overweight and obesity went from 71.2% in 2012 to 72.5% in 2016. However, these differences were not statistically significant (Shama Levy et al., 2016).

5.1.5 *National Epidemiological Surveillance System (SINAVE)*

SINAVE focuses on international epidemiological surveillance and applying measures for the prevention and control of epidemiological problems according to the Official Mexican Standard for Epidemiological Surveillance (Diario Oficial de la Federación, 2013). This is done through coordinated actions of the National Network of Public Health Laboratories (RNLSP), which is integrated by the Institute of Epidemiological Diagnosis and Reference (INDRE) as the network's governing body, the State Public Health Laboratories (LESP) and the Laboratories to Support Epidemiological Surveillance (LAVE). Their participation is essential for the diagnosis of infectious diseases of epidemiological interest, among them dengue, influenza, cholera, tuberculosis, syphilis, HIV and others (INDRE, 2015).

The notification of new cases of diseases subject to epidemiological surveillance is integrated into the Unique Epidemiological Surveillance Information System (SUIVE) (Secretaría de Salud, 2014a), which concentrates the information of 114 surveyed diseases, considered the most relevant to the health status of the population (Dirección General de Epidemiología, 2018) (see section 7.1.4). Furthermore, the surveillance of Health Care Associated Infections (HAIs) is carried out by the Hospital Epidemiological

Surveillance Network (RHOVE), which sets the criteria for the systematic and continuous collection of information generated by each hospital affiliated to RHOVE, according to the Official Mexican Standard for the surveillance, prevention and control of nosocomial infections (Secretaría de Salud, 2009b). During 2015, 61 969 HAIs were reported with an overall incidence rate of 4.7 per 100 discharges (DGE, 2016b).

■ **5.1.6** *Sectoral coordination for public health actions*

Strategies for interinstitutional collaboration with the purpose of improving the population's access to programmes and initiatives have been vigorously implemented in Mexico. One example is the National Health Weeks, which have been in operation for more than 20 years and aim to offer an integrated package of primary care interventions, focusing on immunizations for people under 14 years. The National Health Weeks consist of intensive actions carried out three times a year in which all public NHS institutions participate at the federal, state, municipal and local levels, with the support of other sectors such as education, social development and transportation. Other actions include home visits and installation of vaccination outreach units in high-risk areas and densely populated areas to facilitate access and mass dissemination of health care and information to the population (Secretaría de Salud, 2013a).

Other examples of interinstitutional collaboration involve prevention and health promotion initiatives that are carried out on specific days. Some examples are, 19 October for the International Breast Cancer Day (Instituto Mexicano de la Propiedad Industrial, 2017), 9 August for the National Fight Against Cervical Cancer (Senado de la República, 2016), and 15 February for the International Day of Childhood Cancer (Secretaría de Salud, 2018b). In each instance free early detection and timely treatment campaigns are directed at the public.

■ 5.2 **Patient pathways**

Patient pathways have not been officially regulated, aside from emerging efforts currently being developed through MAIS (see section 5.1). Actual pathways depend on the system's diverse health institutions and enrolment. Pathways also depend on the patient's socioeconomic status, particularly among the non-insured. The agreements for the exchange of highly specialized services among public institutions indicate maximum waiting times for each intervention and, thus, the timing when care should be sought across institutions (Secretaría de Salud, 2012a). Similarly, MoH services can collaborate across state lines to provide care to patients who happen to be outside their normal area of residence or who seek more expeditious care by going to a unit outside it (see section 6.5).

Given the institutional constraints that require long waiting times to receive consultation and access to specialized care as well as deficiencies in the quality of care, the population tends to seek private care or even pay out-of-pocket to access MoH services (see sections 2.1 and 3.4). People affiliated with social insurance institutions or Seguro Popular would have access to primary care services without restrictions, and from there they would be referred to specialized and hospital care services generally provided by the institution itself. In practice, a pattern of mixed public–private health care utilization is frequently observed (see Box 5.1).

BOX 5.1 Model patterns of access to medical care

The following example illustrates a model pattern of access to medical care.

Maria and her husband are employed in the informal sector, so Maria's only option of financial protection was to voluntarily join Seguro Popular. Maria is 40 years old and suffers type 2 diabetes, systemic hypertension, dyslipidaemia, obesity and terminal chronic renal failure that already requires haemodialysis. She goes regularly to an urban health centre belonging to the state health services where a doctor provides her the consultation, a nurse takes samples of blood and urine and a nutritionist gives guidance on diet. The doctor told her that she requires haemodialysis every week, but Seguro Popular does not cover it, so she goes to a private haemodialysis centre where she obtains it at an accessible cost, although it is still expensive. While most of the prescribed medications are dispensed from the health centre, sometimes there are no medications in the pharmacy, and she has to buy the missing medicines from a generic pharmacy out-of-pocket. On one occasion when Maria felt sick, the doctor from the health centre referred her to a Specialized Medical Unit (UNEME), where she was examined by a specialist doctor and asked to continue going there every 3 months to control her diabetes. However, Maria was not able to continue her care at UNEME because it was far away from home and work, and she was tired of waiting for more than an hour to receive care at the health centre. She then began to go to the generic pharmacy more frequently, where a doctor provides care to her for free, prescribes the medicines she needs and always finds them at a low price; she believes that these medicines are more effective than those dispensed at the health centre. On one occasion, Maria had an ulcer on her foot. Immediately, she went to the health centre, where her doctor referred her to an MoH General Hospital an hour away and where they did a small surgery and gave her treatments that saved her foot.

Fortunately, Maria got a salaried job in a self-service store, where she was affiliated with IMSS. They asked her to register with the family medicine unit (UMF) closest to her home, but still 1 hour away, where she took an appointment to receive care. The nurse from the PrevenIMSS care module at the UMF performed laboratory tests and asked her to collect her results in 2 weeks, informing her that she could have diabetes – which of course she already knew. She then requested an appointment by phone to see the family doctor assigned to her, who referred her to do more tests and after 2 weeks confirmed her condition. Maria then began to receive haemodialysis in a private centre which had an agreement with IMSS and where she received all the care free of charge, although it was 2 hours away. Her doctor from the UMF suggested that she follow-up every 2 months and although she was given almost all the medications, she had to wait more than an hour despite having an appointment. She then started going to the pharmacy where she already had confidence that she would receive timely care. She kept going to the UMF from time to time and found out that it was faster for her to request care without an appointment and would receive consultation from a doctor who was available. Through her electronic clinical record, the doctor knew what problems Maria had; however, she always encountered a different doctor and she never had any confidence in them, so she continued alternating her care with the pharmacy doctor. Maria suffered from another foot ulcer, so from the UMF she was referred again to the MoH Zone General Hospital, where her foot was amputated.

A year-and-a-half after getting formal employment at the supermarket, Maria was fired due to a cut in personnel, so she lost her IMSS coverage. Having learned to deal with adversity, she continued going to the pharmacy doctor and to the MoH haemodialysis centre, where she had to cover out-of-pocket expenses. She did not continue working because of her health condition and her disability due to her amputation, as she never received a prosthesis.

■ 5.3 **Primary/ambulatory care**

Primary care operates through institutional provider networks aiming to meet the ambulatory medical care needs of their beneficiaries (see section 4.1.2). Public health institutions (belonging to MoH or social insurance schemes) do not allow a choice of primary care physician; similarly, medical plans in private insurance may limit freedom of choice within closed networks. However, demand for most private sector ambulatory care is guided through personal or physician recommendations with varying degrees of patient choice.

Primary care units have different names depending on the health institutions: health centres, "basic nuclei" and family medicine units, among others (DGIS, 2018a). Each government institution has its own organizational structure and the unit within the state-level government providers is considered the basic nucleus, consisting of a family or general practitioner, a clinical nurse and a public health nurse. Each nucleus is responsible for providing health care to a population in a defined geographical area of up to 500 households and up to 2500 inhabitants. Larger health centres include other health personnel such as social workers, epidemiologists, psychologists, and nutritionists, under the coordination of general practitioners.

Primary care serves as the gateway to the health care system and provides a wide range of services including vaccination, family planning, prenatal care and paediatric care, as well as health promotion outreach such as initiatives to prevent risky behaviours and promote healthy lifestyles (Secretaría de Salud, 2013b). Up to 46.7% (9931) of primary care units in the public sector correspond to fixed establishments located in rural areas and 41% (8736) are located in urban areas. The rest of the units are itinerant services, among which are Fortalecimiento de la Atención Médica Program (formerly Mobile Medical Units) and mobile brigades. These types of units are entrusted with bringing health services closer to people who live in communities whose geographical location is difficult to access. According to the Report of the Observatory of Primary Care Services, in 2012 only 321 primary care units had a clinical laboratory service. Most laboratory services are in urban health centres, although only 13% of these health centres have the service. Similarly, imaging services are found in just 143 primary care units, of which 63% are located in urban health centres (Secretaría de Salud, 2013b).

According to ENSANUT 2012, nearly 40% of the population that used outpatient health services did so in private units, indicating that private care is already an important entry point to the health system (Gutiérrez et al., 2011). Another point of access to primary care services is the Physician in your Home Programme, initially implemented in Mexico City in 2014 and subsequently replicated in other states. In Mexico City, this MoH-funded programme caters to the non-insured, regardless of affiliation to Seguro Popular. Its objective is to provide home care to people who cannot visit a medical unit due to their health conditions. It is aimed at providing medical care to vulnerable populations, mainly the elderly and people with disabilities, and has been extended to pregnant women who have not received prenatal care and terminally ill patients. These health teams are staffed by a doctor and a nurse with the support of social workers, psychologists and dentists; in many cases these personnel are in training. The programme has a permanent 7-days-a-week, 24-hour call centre that offers guidance and allows residents to request a home care visit. The programme provides three categories of home care: mobile pharmacies, mobile laboratory units and the so-called "dental robots" (Secretaría particular del Jefe de Gobierno, 2017). In 2017, the programme serviced more than 200 000 people. However, there is no formal registration system for people in need and no follow-up mechanisms to ensure continuity of care to vulnerable people targeted by the programme (Mir Cervantes et al., 2016). Table 5.1 shows the main strengths and weaknesses of Mexico's primary care services.

5.4 Specialized outpatient care/hospital care

5.4.1 *Specialized outpatient care*

Specialized outpatient care is provided through Specialty Clinics (owned by ISSSTE and MoH), Ambulatory Care Medical Units (owned by IMSS) and private units under different auspices that provide specialty medical and surgical care for patients who do not require hospitalization. There are 100 registered specialized ambulatory care centres in Mexico, of which 64% belong to the public sector (DGIS, 2018b).

The Medical Specialty Units (UNEMES) were created with the objective

TABLE 5.1 Principal strengths and weaknesses of primary care services in Mexico

DIMENSION	STRENGTH	WEAKNESS
Structure	Wide range of services (health promotion, prevention and medical care)	Shortage of health personnel. Insufficiency of supplies for health care
Access	Financial protection with varying scopes of benefits through social insurance and Seguro Popular. Public primary care units located in both urban and rural areas. Itinerant health services for sparsely populated rural areas	Limited working hours. Concentration of care in large units in the case of social insurance. Lack of emergency services in most primary care units
Coordination	Vertical, comprehensive health care networks within each institution	Little integration of health care team in the primary care units and with the specialists of reference hospitals. Lack of horizontal health care networks
Quality of care	Availability of national primary care clinical practice guidelines. Procedures in place to monitor quality of care. Accreditation of primary care facilities within Seguro Popular (until 2019) to enable funding	Low implementation and low adherence to clinical practice guidelines. Deficient continuing education/training. No accreditation by social insurance institutions
Continuity of care	Patients assigned to a family or general physician, with access to clinical records. Referral systems in place	Change of working situation leads to frequent loss of social insurance and hence of family physician. No exchange of clinical records across institutions. Electronic health records only available in IMSS, remain fragmented
Comprehensiveness	Population health needs identified. Community health committees in rural areas carry out coordinated actions with primary care health personnel	Rigid, homogeneous health programmes across diverse institutions and populations

Source: Authors

of bridging primary care and hospital care by providing specialized services for health conditions whose frequency and importance represent a challenge for the health system, such as HIV/AIDS, addictions, chronic diseases and breast cancer, among others (Secretaría de Salud, 2013a). The UNEMES represent 12% of Mexico's total of ambulatory specialized care units (DGIS, 2018b).

The MoH has promoted telehealth or telemedicine to give access to medical care to people who, due to their geographical location, do not have direct access to specialized care. Telemedicine operates in 606 health centres in 21 entities, with which it provides remote care to more than 3 million people. The National Health System institutions – IMSS, ISSSTE, SEDENA and PEMEX – have 4300 professionals who participate in this type of care and, in 2014, 25 051 consultations were given through this service (Secretaría de Salud, 2015c).

5.4.2 *Hospital care*

Hospital care in Mexico is divided across the public and private sectors, with the former catering to acute care needs, particularly for those less well off, while the latter complements services for those better off, offering advanced care and better-quality services. Within the public sector, hospital care is offered by each institution according to its own infrastructure and levels of care, generally distinguishing between general (second level) and high specialty (third level) hospitals (see section 4.1.2). However, many tertiary hospitals also provide a significant proportion of basic specialty services, including normal delivery care. The care of highly complex diseases is funded and provided within MoH through the National Institutes of Health and High Specialty Regional Hospitals, most of which are federal and coordinated by MoH's CINSHAE. IMSS provides specialized hospitalization services in 25 high-specialty medical units, some of which are grouped in medical centres. In the case of ISSSTE, high-specialty care is offered in National Medical Centres. Clinical research is usually undertaken at tertiary care facilities (Saturno et al., 2017).

Private hospitals provide a large range of services according to their size and specialty. The 94 hospitals with more than 49 beds have increasingly focused on supplying diagnostic and treatment medical services through state-of-the-art technology. These hospitals represent 24.3% of all beds and are responsible for 25.1% of all hospital discharges, providing up to 29 diagnostic tests per discharge. In contrast, hospitals with 25 to 49 beds are responsible for 17.6% of discharges and account for 13.6% of beds, but only average up to 13.2 diagnostic tests per discharge. Hospitals with less than 15 beds mainly focus on offering hospitalization services, with only between two and seven diagnostic tests per discharge (González Block et al., 2018b).

> **BOX 5.2** Efforts to improve integration of care
>
> The MoH has implemented cross-institutional integration strategies, most recently in April 2016 through the National Agreement Towards the Universalization of Health Services (*Acuerdo Nacional hacia la Universalización de los Servicios de Salud*) between state, federal and social insurance institutions. The agreement aims to pursue efficiency through complementing capacities across public health institutions and coordinating actions to increase effective access. The agreement includes only selected high specialty services such as magnetic resonance or intensive care for specific conditions. The high-specialty services exchange agreements, particularly the emergency obstetric care programme, are framed as universalizing access, regardless of the person's insurance status. The plan envisages that in the future patients will be able to choose the institution they prefer, according to needs and preferences. The electronic clinical record has also been supported by diverse institutions to facilitate universal coverage. While a national standard ensures interoperability, implementation has been slow and limited to hospital care, except in IMSS.

5.4.3 *Evaluation of the quality of acute medical care*

Accreditation is limited to MoH primary care and hospital units participating in Seguro Popular and is applied periodically as a method of external evaluation to determine if it meets standards of capacity, quality and safety (DGCES, 2018). Of the 14 332 MoH primary care units, 9801 (68.4%) have been accredited (see section 2.5.6). With respect to the hospital units, of the 751 MoH hospitals, 510 have current accreditation for CAUSES and 538 also have accreditation for at least one intervention funded by FPGC (DGIS, 2018b).

Voluntary accreditation by the General Health Board through SiNaCEAM has been attained by 282 hospitals, most of which (197) are private. SiNaCEAM has accredited four of 27 IMSS high-specialty hospitals, four of 12 National Institutes of Health and only eight MoH general hospitals. The majority of PEMEX hospitals are accredited, being the institution with the highest per capita health expenditure (Consejo General de Salud, 2015) (see section 3.2.1).

In addition, DGCES also coordinates the National System for Quality of Care Indicators (INDICAS), a tool that monitors medical and nursing quality indicators in MoH primary care health units and hospitals, including patient-reported process measures such as satisfaction with the timeliness of care and the information provided, the supply of medications, the quality of treatment received, waiting times and surgical deferment (Secretaría de Salud, 2016a). The indicator of perceived quality during the 2003–2017 period shows very high approval ratings overall, with primary care exceeding the expected minimum qualification standard of 95% and hospital care showing indicators above 90% for emergency care and well above 95% for nursing care (Figure 5.1). An evaluation of the INDICAS system found these results surprisingly consistent across indicators, as well as inconsistent with those of other information sources such as ENSANUT (Saturno et al., 2014).

FIG. 5.1 Perceived quality indicators, National Health System, 2003–2017

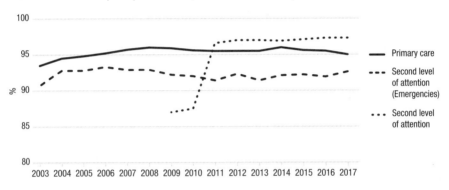

Source: DGCES Dirección General de Calidad y Educación en Salud, Secretaría de Salud (2018)

5.4.4 *Day care*

The public health system does not provide day care services for people with health problems, although these units are available in the private sector. The Official Mexican Standard for Day Care Centres defines day care centres as establishments for the care of the elderly and for the creative and productive occupation of their leisure time (Secretaría de Salud, 1999). Although they may directly provide medical attention or use external health personnel for prevention or detection of specific health problems, the main objective of these centres is to provide general care or social support during daytime hours.

Patients who require short-term hospital care (e.g. day surgeries) are usually treated in general or specialty hospitals through specific services according to the type of pathologies and diagnosis. The most frequent reason for short-stay care is surgery. Both public and private health institutions have short-stay surgery programmes (less than 3-days' hospitalization) that account for the majority of their surgical discharges (IMSS, 2005).

Some hospitals provide services for short-stay care for conditions that require treatments in non-surgical hospital areas. Examples are the Department of Hematology-Oncology of the Children's Hospital of Mexico Federico Gómez, the main specialized care centre for children with cancer, which provides outpatient chemotherapy therapies and includes a play room for children, where they can stay with their parents during daytime hours before and after their treatment session (Hospital Infantil de México Federico Gómez, 2012).

The IMSS has implemented a Centre for Social Care of the Health of Older Adults (CAMOHM), which provides day care to people over 60 with activities aimed at stimulating their physical, mental (cognitive), emotional and social spheres; likewise, the programme provides gerontology care by evaluating patients' physical and mental functioning (Perez Cuevas et al., 2015). However, this service is only granted in a single establishment in Mexico City, so its benefit is very limited. In addition, the National Institute for Older Persons (INAPAM) has seven units providing day residency in Mexico City, consisting of temporary daytime stays for people 60 and older, who are poor but functionally independent or who find themselves alone and want to socialize with people of the same age. Residents are provided with medical, psychological, social work, occupational and recreational activities, as well as with meals (INAPAM, 2014).

5.5 **Emergency care**

Emergency care is provided through emergency services in both public and private hospitals. People with life-threatening problems, or their caregivers, can legally go to the emergency department of any hospital or request an ambulance service and prehospital medical care. Public health services provide ambulance services at no cost, and the Red Cross offers emergency ambulance services at low cost. Private ambulances vary according to the services they provide. There is a 911 number for emergencies which directs calls to the nearest emergency services unit, regardless of the institutional coverage of the person in need. Each of the emergency units (first responders) has a geolocation so the operator can identify the nearest unit for referral. This system has access to more than 3000 first responders (police, paramedics and firemen) located in 194 call centres countrywide; operators know the emergency medical protocols and are trained to perform crisis intervention. In addition, they can provide telephone first aid, which increases the quality of service and the chances of survival of those who need help (Secretaría de Salud, 2011).

There are multiple agencies and institutions that provide emergency prehospital care services in Mexico, such as government agencies (civil protection, firefighters, rescue squadrons and medical emergency responders in some states, etc.), the Mexican Red Cross and various private companies that provide care for privately insured patients (Fraga et al., 2010). Public hospitals and private hospitals operate emergency services 24 hours a day, attended by general practitioners and specialists in medical emergencies. There are also specialists in basic areas such as paediatrics, obstetrics and gynaecology, internal medicine, general surgery and orthopaedics.

In the particular case of obstetric emergencies and with the objective of reducing maternal mortality, public sector institutions established a General Agreement for Interinstitutional Collaboration for the Care of Obstetric Emergencies. This instrument allows any pregnant woman who shows signs of distress to go to the nearest IMSS, ISSSTE or MoH medical unit, regardless of their affiliation. If the medical unit has the required clinical capacity to attend the obstetric emergency, it must accept and provide the necessary medical care at no cost to the woman and her newborn. If the unit does not have the clinical capacity, they are responsible for transferring the woman to a unit that does, also at no cost. Once the mother and the newborn are discharged, the institutions can claim payment according to the patient's institutional affiliation (Secretaría de Salud, 2012b). Payments across institutions may be delayed or not be reimbursed in cases of care for uninsured women not affiliated to Seguro Popular, although affiliation is possible within MoH hospitals at the time when health care is demanded.

■ 5.6 **Pharmaceutical care**

The regulation and governance of the pharmaceutical industry is described in section 2.6, while the analysis of financing is discussed in section 3. In this section, we describe the production, distribution and supply of medicines.

■ **5.6.1** *Pharmaceutical policy*

Mexico does not have an integrated pharmaceutical policy to follow the recommendations of the World Health Organization in terms of the definition and prioritization of medium- and long-term governmental objectives for the pharmaceutical sector (WHO, 2001). In 2005, foundations were established for a policy through a framework document that included chapters on safety, efficacy and quality of medicines, availability and access, and innovation and competitiveness of the pharmaceutical industry, with specific strategies and lines of action; however, these recommendations have not been fully implemented (Secretaría de Salud, 2005).

Since 2005, there have been numerous attempts to reform pharmaceutical policies. The sectoral health programmes in the government periods of 2007–2012 and 2013–2018 have included strategies and action plans to improve access to medicines, some of which have been taken forward (González Pier, 2008; Dresser et al., 2008; Wirtz, Dresser & Heredia Pi, 2013; González Pier & Barraza, 2011). Although a voluntary notification of adverse drug reactions programme began in 1989 and the National Centre for Pharmacovigilance was created in 2001, its actions are incipient and there is a lack of systematization in reports by health professionals, so that voluntary notifications of adverse events are limited. To address these problems, new pharmacovigilance regulations were enacted in 2018 applicable to all agencies in the health system, including drug distributors and retailers to strengthen the notification of adverse events and reactions produced by medications, as well as the reporting of drug safety in clinical studies (Diario Oficial de la Federación, 2017a; COFEPRIS, 2018).

■ 5.6.2 *Pharmaceutical market*

Mexico's pharmaceutical industry is the second largest in Latin America and represents almost 0.5% of GDP, with ongoing increases in production and consumption. In 2015, a total of 742 pharmaceutical companies were in operation, the main ones being foreign corporations, mostly from the United States (Secretaría de Economía, 2016). A total of 306 national companies are in operation, mostly producing generics (Table 5.2).

The National Association of Pharmaceutical Manufacturers – an organization of pharmaceutical entrepreneurs – represents 28 pharmaceutical firms funded predominantly through Mexican capital that produce 60% of their medicines for public health institutions and the rest for the private sector (ANAFAM, 2018). According to INEGI, the country's largest volume of drug production corresponds to antibiotics at 23% of the total, followed by digestive system and metabolism medications (12.3%), analgesics (8.6%) and supplements (8.1%) (INEGI, 2017b).

TABLE 5.2 National firms of allopathic, homeopathic or herbal medicines with a health licence

TYPE OF PRODUCT	NUMBER OF FIRMS
Allopathic	280
Herbalist	3
Homeopathic	1
More than one category (homeopathic + herbalist; herbalist + allopathic)	9
Medicinal gases	13
Total	**306**

Source: COFEPRIS (2016a)

The pharmaceutical market differs in the public and private sectors, with patent medicines being mainly for consumption through the private sector and generics (with approved bioequivalence) (Gutiérrez et al., 2011) addressing public sector needs. An analysis conducted by the Mexican Health Foundation – a private Mexican NGO – showed that most of the volume of pharmaceutical sales consists of generics in any form, and only 1.5% consists of patented medications (Funsalud, 2012). In another study, 10% of retail sales were reported as being "similar" drugs (Gómez Dantés, 2011), which are the same generic products in different guises.

In the public sector, IMSS represents 45% of the total public market for medicines (Moreno, López & García 2016). Since 2006, IMSS established consolidated purchasing of medicines, with the objective of obtaining lower prices for all its hospitals and clinics, a practice that now includes purchases for other public health institutions at the federal and state levels. In the period 2017–2018, an estimated 49 institutions participated in concentrated purchases through IMSS, reportedly saving more than 3 billion pesos (US$ 150 million) (IMSS, 2018). The procurement of medicines in the public health sector is based on the Basic Table and Catalogue of Medicines, which regulates the supplies in this area and to which all public institutions must comply. The list includes 14 092 drug codes and a total of 2816 generic drugs (Diario Oficial de la Federación, 2017b).

5.6.3 *Distribution of medicines*

Wholesale distributors are primarily concentrated in three large companies that control, store and transport pharmaceutical products to pharmacy chains and private health establishments. There are also specialized distributors for the public sector, focusing on government procurement. In 2014, there were more than 80 000 pharmacies, of which 86% were independent (69 787), 10% corresponded to chain pharmacies (8387) and 4% were installed in self-service stores (3105) (González Block et al., 2018b). Retail establishments are represented by different organizations addressing pharmacy chains, independent community pharmacies and pharmacies in self-service stores (Table 5.3).

TABLE 5.3 Main organizations grouping drug dispensers in Mexico

ORGANIZATION	CHARACTERISTIC
National Association of Pharmacies of Mexico (ANAFARMEX)	15 000 independent pharmacies and chains
National Union of Pharmacy Entrepreneurs (UNEFARM)	More than 5000 pharmacies belonging to 28 pharmaceutical groups
National Association of Drug Distributors (ANADIM)	Groups 23 companies with six regional distributors and 17 pharmacy chains with 7725 pharmacies
National Association of Regional Pharmaceutical Companies (ANEFAR)	17 active partners with 400 pharmacies
Pharmacies "Similar"	Four companies with more than 6000 pharmacies

Note: Information obtained from organizations' websites

Source: Authors

5.6.4 *Dispensing medications*

With regard to the dispensing of pharmaceuticals, social insurance institutions perform this function within their medical establishments through their own pharmacies at no cost. Likewise, MoH facilities provided medicines free of charge to the population covered by Seguro Popular according to CAUSES (CNPSS, 2018a). However, access to medication is still incomplete in practice. ENSANUT 2012 reported that only 65.2% of those who received a prescription for medication in any public ambulatory medical unit obtained all prescriptions in the same place of care, with variation in the dispensation between IMSS (86.1%) and the MoH (63.7%). The supply of medications within the pharmacies with an adjacent physician (CAF) was 74.6% (Gutiérrez et al., 2011).

5.6.5 *Introduction of new molecules*

In response to Mexico's expanding national market for medicines, the approval of new molecules protected by patent is growing, given both the increased market access push by the pharmaceutical industry and the acceleration of the approval process by COFEPRIS and the General Health Council. However, the rate of inclusion of new patent medicines in basic public health institutions' frameworks has decreased considerably. While in 2009, a total of 49 and 58 new drugs were included in the lists of IMSS and ISSSTE, respectively, these collapsed to 0 and 1 in 2014, although they had a slight rebound in 2015, reaching 13 and 5, respectively. IMSS only accepted 21% of the applications it received, and ISSSTE, 8%, mainly due to budget limitations (González Block et al., 2018b). The largest number of innovative molecules in the market is limited, therefore, to consumption in the private market, which increases the pressure on out-of-pocket expenses and private insurance.

5.6.6 *Generic drugs*

The federal government has made the promotion of generic medicines a priority since at least the end of the 1990s. However, in just the last 6 years COFEPRIS has approved 590 additional generic products, of which 43 active substances are offered with prices at 70% lower than their brand counterparts. The new generics have expanded the range of options for over 20 therapeutic classes such as antibiotics, analgesics and treatments for diseases such as diabetes, cancer and hypertension (Presidencia de la República, 2018). However, the growth of the generic drug market has not been as rapid as might have been expected. According to a COFECE study, four out of every 10 drugs that have lost their patent in Mexico lack competition for a generic drug (Comisión Federal de Competencia Económica, 2017). On average more than 2 years elapse before molecules that lose their patents enter the generics market, compared with other countries where this transition is immediate or only takes a few months. In addition, for each drug that loses its patent and enters the generic market, just 2.8 competitors participate in Mexico, compared with 10.1 in the United States. The price reduction observed after 2 years due to the introduction of competition is only 20%, compared with 40% in the European Union. This translates into a loss for Mexican households, which are spending more than $ 2.5 billion additional pesos per year – 0.54% of out-of-pocket spending on health – that could be avoided with greater competition.

There are several factors that inhibit the competition in generics. These include the issuance of several patents on the same active substance, the legal defence of patents, the lack of coordination regarding information on patents and sanitary registration, the lack of transparency in regard to deadlines and the subsequent management of applications for the registration of new molecules and for extensions, and the lack of regulations mandating physicians to prescribe the generic example, as opposed to the brand name.

■ **5.6.7** *The integration of prescription and dispensation*

A recent challenge that increasingly affects both the prescription and dispensation of medicines is the growing proliferation of medical consulting rooms adjacent to pharmacies (CAF). This business model emerged at the end of the 1990s to strengthen the prestige of generic drugs. The model is based on a low-cost care strategy offered by general practitioners who are hired under varying incentive schemes tied to the sale of medicines. This strategy was strengthened in 2010 when a regulation came into force to demand the presentation of a medical prescription as a condition for the sale of antibiotics, medicines which are in high demand in private pharmacies.

Recent reports have identified that by 2015, the number of CAFs had risen to 15 000 in chain pharmacies or independent pharmacies (Díaz Portillo et al., 2017). The potential implications of this trend, which has gained increasingly popular acceptance due to the convenience of shorter waiting times and lower consultation costs (Funsalud, 2014), include a lack of supervision of the quality of care provided in these facilities, with the risk of inappropriate prescriptions and possible conflicts of interest with pharmacy owners who are incentivized to promote the sale of their products. However, an analysis of the retail sales data in kilograms of antibiotics between 2007 and 2012 reported that the estimated defined daily dose (DDD) per 1000/ days decreased among Mexicans in that period by 29.2% (Santa Ana et al., 2013), possibly as an effect of the 2010 prescription regulation.

5.7 **Rehabilitation and intermediate care**

5.7.1 *Rehabilitation*

The rehabilitation of patients with disabilities is mainly provided by public and private non-profit institutions. The MoH's National Institute of Rehabilitation is a high-specialty centre that includes rehabilitation medicine with hospital care, extramural surgery and outpatient care as well as the specialties of orthopaedics, audiology and otorhinolaryngology and a burns care centre. Other national institutes such as the General Hospital of Mexico and the Children's Hospital of Mexico also have rehabilitation services. The DIF serves patients in need of rehabilitation without social insurance through the Prevention, Rehabilitation and Social Inclusion Programme for Persons with Disabilities and their families. The DIF operates rehabilitation centres that seek to improve patients' quality of life through comprehensive rehabilitative care and the promotion of education, and labour and social inclusion (Sistema Nacional DIF, 2016).

In the social insurance subsystem, IMSS has the largest network of rehabilitation care in Mexico, with three highly specialized medical units, a general hospital and 131 rehabilitation services subunits operating in hospitals of different levels of care. In the past decade, 49 rehabilitation services centres have been installed in family medicine units (primary care clinics) throughout the country, which include a doctor specializing in physical medicine and rehabilitation, four physical therapists, a social worker and a nurse (Guzmán González, 2016). Other social insurance institutions (namely ISSSTE and SEDENA) offer rehabilitation care in high-specialty units with hospital services and outpatient services in physical medicine and rehabilitation.

The rehabilitation provided by private institutions of social assistance has made important growth, being one of the health areas with greater social mobilization. The Association for the Support of People with Cerebral Palsy (APAC) provides specialized care to people with this condition and related disabilities through rehabilitation, medical assistance and psychological care, specialized education, training for work and support for their social inclusion (Asociación Pro Personas con Parálisis Cerebral, 2018). The Telethon Foundation's Teletón Children's System (SIT) operates 22 Rehabilitation and Childhood Inclusion Telethon Centres (CRIT) in the country, offering care to more than 27 000 children up to 18 years of age who struggle with neuromusculoskeletal disabilities, by providing comprehensive rehabilitation services based on a family-centred model (Fundación Teletón, 2015).

5.7.2 *Intermediate care*

MoH has implemented a network of medical facilities called Specialized Medical Units in Chronic Diseases (UNEMES-EC) tasked with providing intermediate care aimed at reducing hospitalizations. These facilities provide care to patients with type 2 diabetes, hypertension, obesity, dyslipidaemias and metabolic syndromes that were not brought under control during the first level of care. Services are provided through a multidisciplinary team consisting of a specialist physician, who also coordinates the unit, supported by nurses, social workers, psychologists and nutritionists to help reduce current saturation rates and operating costs in hospitals. The objective is to reduce complications associated with these conditions through its network of 100 units, operating in 29 states. Preliminary evaluations of this initiative has reported improvement in some metabolic indicators with respect to those reported at the first level of care (Contreras Loya, Reding Beltran & Gómez Dantés, 2013).

■ 5.8 **Long-term care**

Mexico lacks a system to provide permanent long-term care services for people living with chronic conditions, disability or loss of functionality due to advanced age, whether in hospital care centres, residences or community care. Specific programmes are available in some institutions that include some aspects of these health care services, such as those of INAPAM, which has shelters that provide comprehensive assistance to older adults who lack family support or economic resources, allowing them to cover their basic needs and be independent. There are six shelters (four in Mexico City and two in cities in Mexico's interior) which offer permanent accommodation and balanced feeding services, medical, psychological, geriatric supervision, occupational and recreational therapy. Those seeking to enter a shelter must be more than 60 years old, without other means of support and fall within socioeconomic, medical and psychological criteria that meets compliance requirements for admission (INAPAM, 2014).

At the private level, long-term care is offered in residences mainly for the elderly or people requiring home care that includes daily professional care, intermediate care, part-time professional care and custody and not necessarily professional assistance. Geriatric residences usually have an intervention programme (geriatric and permanent nursing care, nutrition services and recreational activities) and can also function as day centres. In 2015, a register of institutions for the care of older adults reported 2692 facilities for the care of the elderly, including clubs, shelters and day residences throughout the country (INAPAM, 2016). There is also private care in the form of insurance such as homes or home care, either with one or both services. The periods of care guaranteed by the policies generally vary between 3 and 10 years, including medical care or assistance from other professionals.

There are numerous providers of home care services for the care of the chronically ill, elderly people with functional impairment, people with severe disability or terminal illness. Although there is no formal census of paid caregivers, in 2016 INEGI reported close to 286 000 people dedicated to this task, of which 96.7% are women, with 38% working in establishments and 62% attending to patients in the latter's domiciles, with no remuneration for this job. Carers are predominantly young (two thirds between 15 and 39 years old), with average- to mid-level high schooling, who work in establishments, while caregivers working in private homes have mostly average- or elementary-level schooling. The average income of paid caregivers is 24.3 pesos per hour (US$ 1.21 estimated at 20 pesos for US$ 1) and the number of average hours worked is 38.5 per week (INEGI, 2017c).

5.9 **Care by informal caregivers**

Informal care is defined as support provided free of charge in the family environment for people in need of assistance to carry out their daily activities due to loss of physical, mental or intellectual capacity (dependent persons). Informal care represents a high social and economic value that is little recognized in Mexico and is without regulation or support.

A 2012 Labor and Social Co-responsibility Survey (ELCOS) showed that the short-term care of temporary patients, as well as the long-term care of people with permanent limitations, is carried out by a member of the same household in more than 80% of cases; approximately 70% of these carers are women. Half of the cases of care for short-term patients are the responsibility of a single person, while long-term care for people with permanent limitations was divided between two people in 40% of cases (Inmujeres, 2012). The care and support for short-term patients, chronically ill people and people with some physical or mental limitation represented 7.5% of Mexico's GDP, according to the Satellite Account of Unpaid Home Work in Mexico 2016 (INEGI, 2016c).

Public programmes to support informal carers are scarce. The ISSSTE has a Support Course for Informal Caregivers of Aging Persons, available to all public on its web portal tailored to self-learning about the basic care of the elderly in the home and in the care of the caregivers (ISSSTE, 2014).

5.10 **Palliative care**

The emergence of palliative care as a topic of public concern in the Mexican public health agenda is of recent origin. In 2009, a section for palliative care for terminally ill patients was included in the General Health Law (Diario Oficial de la Federación, 2009), while the first Official Mexican Standard for the Care of Terminally Ill Patients Through Palliative Care was published in 2014. In 2016, an agreement declaring comprehensive palliative care management schemes as compulsory was made, followed by the issuing of the Comprehensive Management Guide for Palliative Care in the Pediatric Patient (Diario Oficial de la Federación, 2014 & 2016).

Despite these efforts, WHO has classified Mexico in the group of countries with limited provision of palliative care, given the disparate service standards, insufficient support that frequently depends on donors, and limited availability of morphine with respect to the size of the population. Paediatric palliative care was rated by WHO at an even lower level of development, for its stage of organization, personnel training and incipient capacity for the provision of services (Connor & Sepulveda, 2015).

There is no national public policy to coordinate the care of patients who require palliative care in terms of service networks and levels of care. Palliative care has been implemented through localized initiatives in some highly specialized hospitals and public hospitals and there are no records of the number of facilities with such services. According to COFEPRIS, there are 71 primary-level care palliative care services in Mexico, 34 secondary-care level and 10 tertiary-level (COFEPRIS, 2016) (Table 5.4). Additionally, four multilevel services providing care for public dependencies were reported, a day centre in the National Institute of Cancerology and 14 teams of hospice volunteers, all of them private and non-profit (Pastrana et al., 2012).

TABLE 5.4 Palliative care services in Mexico, 2012

LEVEL OF CARE	SERVICES	NUMBER (PROVIDER)	CHARACTERISTICS
First level	Hospice type residence	7 (OSCs)	Psychologists, social workers, volunteers and family members
	Home care	47 teams (IMSS and OSCs)	Doctors and specialized nurses and psychologists
	Community centre (Home care)	17 teams (Mexico City Government and OSCs)	General practitioners and trained nurses
Second level	Hospitalization	34 (State general hospitals, university, state oncology centres and ISSSTE)	Units with doctors specialized in palliative care, nurses and psychology services, thanatology, nutrition, social work, respiratory therapy, rehabilitation and in some cases pain therapy
Third level	Hospitalization of high-specialty	10 (National Institutes of Health of the MoH, IMSS & ISSSTE)	Exclusive units for palliative care with multi-professional specialists and in some cases including pain clinics

OSC: Civil society organization

Source: Pastrana et al. (2012)

One of the limitations for palliative care is the insufficient availability of opioid medications for the treatment of pain. In 2016, COFEPRIS took steps to address this limitation by conferring with medical associations, health institutions, the pharmaceutical industry and its distributors and pharmacies, about the public need and demand for such medications, which led to the establishment of a Rapid Action Group. By the end of 2017, COFEPRIS signed an agreement with the United Nations Office on Drugs and Crime (UNODC) called the "Access to Controlled Substances for Medical Purposes", which employs the slogan "Access without Excess" and aims to promote patient access to controlled medications in the context of their palliative care (COFEPRIS, 2017).

However, the restrictions and protocols required to receive an opioid prescription continue to limit access. Among them, the need for an obligatory special prescription with a bar code identifying the medicine as a narcotic and an onerous procedure required by COFEPRIS to obtain it (COFEPRIS, 2016b). Of 163 000 general practitioners and registered specialists in the country (see section 4.2.1), only 3664 have the capacity to issue specialized prescriptions (2.24%).

■ 5.11 **Mental health**

Mental health in Mexico is a growing problem (see sections 1.4.2 and 1.4.3), one in five individuals has at least one mental disorder at a time in their life (de la Fuente, 2014). However, there is limited investment in mental health care. During 2017 the budget allocated for mental health was only 2586 million pesos, just over $ 1.00 per capita (Center for Economic and Budgetary Research, 2017). In addition, it has been described that 80% of the mental health budget is used for the operation of psychiatric hospitals, leaving only 20% to finance the rest of the mental health services network, with a critically short supply of community mental health services (Berenzon Gorn, 2013; Oficina de Información Científica y Tecnológica para el Congreso de la Unión, 2018).

Mexico's current mental health policy is based on the Miguel Hidalgo Model of Mental Health Care (Programme for Specific Action for Mental Health 2013–2018, Secretaría de Salud). This reform, also implemented in Spain and Italy, follows three principles:

- The strengthening of initiatives that increase the public awareness of mental health as well as community care, promote outpatient services and reduce the need for hospitalization as much as possible.
- Hospitalization, when required, should be short stay, in psychiatric units ideally incorporated in general hospitals.
- The existence of psychosocial rehabilitation and social reintegration services that reintegrate the person with mental illness into their community.

These principles aim to reduce hospitalizations as much as possible, re-admissions and definitively eradicate long-term stays, giving patients better care and at the same time a higher quality of life.

Current efforts in the Mexican health system are aimed at the reorganization of services with the aim of replacing prolonged stays in psychiatric hospitals with assistance through a network of interrelated community services. These include primary care, outpatient care in psychiatric units in general hospitals and support for people with mental disorders who live with their families or in subsidized housing. Likewise, these reforms propose to add to the clinical–pharmacological process characteristic of in-hospital treatment, psychosocial rehabilitation programmes (therapeutic walks, protected workshops, etc.) focused on the reintegration of the patient into their community.

The 2006 Mexican Declaration on Psychiatric Restructuring was signed by the state secretaries of health and other authorities. This declaration represents a milestone in the political support for a new way of conceiving of mental health care in Mexico. One outcome was the establishment of the Hospital Transition Villas in six states (State of Mexico, Jalisco, Tamaulipas, Hidalgo, Durango and Oaxaca) as a means to protect the rights of people with disabilities and to contribute to their integral development and full inclusion (Secretaría de Salud, 2013c). Seguro Popular financed seven mental health interventions in CAUSES: attention deficit disorder with hyperactive component, depression, affective disorders such as bipolar affective disorder, anxiety disorders and psychotic disorders such as schizophrenia (CNPSS, 2018a). However, many patients with mental health disorders covered by Seguro Popular still struggled with difficulties in the referral process and the confirmation of the validation of payments.

Mexico suffers from insufficient mental health human resources. For decades, most mental health resources were concentrated in psychiatric hospitals (OPS, 2013). In 2016, 4393 psychiatrists practised in Mexico, a rate of just 3.68 psychiatrists per 100 000 inhabitants. In addition, there is a poor distribution of these specialists across the country, with around 60% practising in the three main cities of Mexico (Heinze, Chapa & Carmona-Huerta, 2016). In an effort to address the country's mental health needs, numbers of specialized mental health personnel have increased at the primary care level of the community. In 2012, 42 UNEME mental health centres were established, the so-called Integrated Mental Health Centres (UNEMES-CISAME). These units are available in 20 states and provide outpatient care with a comprehensive model, close to the community, via basic multidisciplinary teams consisting of a psychiatrist, a clinical psychologist, a psychologist with specialty in psychotherapy, a social worker and nursing staff (OPS, 2013).

There are a total of 38 psychiatric hospitals, of which 34 are housed under the MoH and four under IMSS (Secretaría de Salud, 2013c). In the most recent evaluation of Mexico's mental health services it was found that even though the number of outpatient services has increased, the psychiatric hospital remains the centre of mental health care, providing care for close to half of patients receiving care for mental health conditions (Berenzon et al., 2013). In relation to the length of inpatient stay, patients were hospitalized for an average of 24 days; however, 38% remained in psychiatric hospitals for a period of 5 or more years.

Mental health care for disaster situations and for highly violent communities is also in short supply. The Mental Health Action Programme has identified this need at least since 2001 (Secretary of Health, 2001). However, information is lacking to assess mental health services in these contexts. Civil society organizations such as Doctors Without Borders provide mental health care to people affected by violence through four projects implemented in Mexico located in Tabasco, Veracruz, Mexico City, Tamaulipas and Guerrero. However, the integration of specific government programmes for the care of the population affected by this problem is required (Médicos Sin Fronteras, 2019). The situation and response to the mental health of migrants is addressed in section 2.7.5 on cross-border health.

◼ 5.12 **Dental care**

Dental health is provided primarily by private services (see section 4.2.2). Public services have dental offices in ambulatory care units, urban and rural, that provide limited services to their patients. In the private sector, providers are remunerated mainly through direct payments by the patient and, to a lesser extent, through private medical insurance contracted by the insured or his or her employer.

In the public sector, the human resources contracted to provide oral health care services represent less than 20% of all dentists in Mexico (see section 4.2.2), while public institutions grapple with high volumes of patients and short consultation times per dentist, ranging from 20 minutes in ISSSTE to 45 minutes in MoH units (Secretaría de Salud, 2013d). However, Mexico has oral health policies such as the School Health Programme as well as preventive health regulations for the iodization and fluoridation of salt. Public sector ambulatory care units monitor dental health at the different stages of life, and monitoring oral health is also integrated into the National System of Health Records and the Epidemiological Surveillance System of Oral Pathologies (SIVEPAB), with 413 units throughout the country that provide epidemiological information on the most important oral problems. All these initiatives are regulated by the Official Mexican Standard for the Prevention and Control of Oral Diseases and are applied mainly in the public sector (Secretaría de Salud, 2014b).

◼ 5.13 **Complementary and alternative medicine**

The MoH recognizes the importance of traditional medicine understood as a set of medical systems rooted in health and disease knowledge accumulated by the different Indigenous peoples of Mexico throughout their histories. It also recognizes complementary or alternative medicine, referring to various therapeutic models that are not part of the Mexican health care tradition and that are not integrated into its prevailing health system.

The Directorate for Traditional Medicine and Intercultural Development (DMTDI), housed within DGPLADES, recognizes the cultural diversity of the country's Mestizo and Indigenous populations and to the emergence of new paradigms in the definition of health care programmes. From 2002 to

2012, Specific Action Programmes (PAE) were published in recognition of Traditional Medicine and Complementary Health Care Systems, and which promote the generation of knowledge about traditional and complementary medicine as well as its safe use (Secretaría de Salud, 2007b). However, during the 2013–2018 period, no PAE was issued to give continuity to these actions.

In Mexico, more than 125 different complementary medicine therapies are practised in 20 states, with a prevalence of use ranging from 18% to 75% and an average of 45%. Among the main advances in complementary medicine is the inclusion of a legal basis for the practice of various complementary therapies in the current regulatory framework. Such is the case of acupuncture, regulated by the Official Mexican Regulation of Health Services for the Practise of Human Acupuncture and Related Methods (Secretaría de Salud, 2012b). Likewise, since 1997, the General Health Law has recognized the existence of allopathic, homeopathic and herbal medicines and these are acknowledged in the Herbalist Pharmacopoeia of the United Mexican States (Secretaría de Salud, 2007b).

As of 2006, homeopathy and acupuncture clinics have been incorporated into the model of medical units of the health infrastructure master plan (PMI) and health cards for the provision of these services began to be distributed. Currently, homeopathy and acupuncture are integrated into numerous MoH, ISSSTE, SEMAR and university hospitals. In addition, there are 15 Integral Hospitals that specialize in traditional medicine and strengthened by intercultural elements, 14 of which are in the state of Puebla and one in Nayarit (Secretaría de Salud, 2014c). Additionally, the DMTDI has recently dedicated efforts to the implementation of vertical delivery in several hospitals in the country (Campos Navarro, Peña Sánchez & Paulo Maya, 2017).

DMTDI's strategies are particularly apparent in traditional, complementary and intercultural medicine programmes, most notably in the states of Querétaro, Hidalgo, Puebla and Veracruz. Less influence has been observed in the states with the greatest Indigenous presence such as Michoacán, Guerrero, Oaxaca and Chiapas. Furthermore, institutional programmes and strategies are contradictory and ambiguous (Campos Navarro, Peña Sánchez & Paulo Maya, 2017). Given Mexico's large Indigenous population (see section 1.1), it is of concern that public policy initiatives related to the provision of health services through intercultural programmes are still incipient.

6

Principal health reforms

■ Chapter summary

- National health policy and reforms since 1983 have aimed to integrate the segmented health system into a more coherent whole to attain greater equity and efficiency.
- The constitutional reform of 1983 introduced the right to health protection and the 2011 amendment to Article 1 recognizes health as a human right. However, the MoH has limited capacity and authority to influence policy across health programmes for the uninsured, particularly so for social insurance institutions and the private sector.
- The General Health Law defines the National Health System based on the right to health protection rather than the right to the attainment of the highest possible levels of health for all. The National Health System is, therefore, less an integrated whole and more a set of coordinated measures across federal institutions and states as well as across the private sector.
- Among the most important reforms since 2000 were the 2003 establishment of SPSS, involving the federal and state governments, and the Strategy for Portability and Convergence, implemented from 2006 and involving mostly federal institutions. In 2014, a reform was implemented to increase SPSS accountability.

- There is general agreement today for the need for a constitutional reform to provide the MoH with greater powers to formulate policy across all public and private health institutions and to de-link health service access from the labour market.
- The new government of Andrés Manuel López Obrador, in place since December 2018, promised to focus on combating corruption and poverty and aims towards the establishment of a Universal Public Health System integrating MoH and social insurance institutions.
- To this end, the new government substituted the SPSS with a Policy for Free Health Services and Medicines and with the Institute for Health for Wellbeing (INSABI).

6.1 The System for Social Protection in Health

In the transition to an opposition-led federal government in December 2000, health policy in Mexico aimed to establish universal health coverage by strengthening funding and services for the self-employed and informal sector workers segment of the labour market, the latter comprising over half of Mexico's active labour force. These two groups were to be gradually incorporated on a voluntary basis into Seguro Popular, SPSS's operational arm. A legal reform earmarked new funding for the uninsured that aimed to protect them from catastrophic health expenditures while transforming incentives from the supply side to the demand side, and separating financing from provision. The administration of President López Obrador substituted SPSS for a policy of universal access to services and free medicines still under implementation, eliminating demand-side funding and reverting to historical funding through INSABI.

SPSS did not aim to integrate the various segments of the health system. This would have required transforming the last enclaves of corporatist health services, a formidable task for an opposition government and a nascent democracy that had to demonstrate quick wins. The objective was, rather, to consolidate the weakest segment in the corporatist system, planting the seeds for major change in the future.

Consolidation of the National Health System through SPSS meant raising the uninsured segment to the level of benefits provided by IMSS in at least two broad stages: in 2012, all the uninsured would gain entry to Seguro Popular, which would offer a comprehensive though still limited set of benefits compared with those afforded to IMSS beneficiaries. Thereafter, the package of services would be increased to eventually achieve equity and to open up the possibility for the integration of health institutions beyond labour market segmentation.

Seguro Popular was implemented through the enactment of SPSS, whereby Congress allocated funding according to voluntary registration with Seguro Popular. SPSS included a tripartite funding arrangement following social insurance schemes so that it could eventually be assimilated into mainstream funding channels (Ibarra et al., 2013) (see sections 2.1.9 and 3.3.1). The government share was contributed by both the federal and state governments while the federal government's share was equivalent to that contributed by the employers in IMSS. Individuals contributed according to income, with exemptions for low-income population up to income decile IV.

■ 6.2 **Financial impact of SPSS**

The SPSS emerged from the policy objective to overcome five financial imbalances that markedly limited the equity and efficiency of public health institutions at the beginning of the new century (Table 6.1). The first imbalance was that of insufficient spending on health. At only 5.0% of GDP, health spending was widely considered to be insufficient to meet the health needs of the population. The second imbalance was related to excessive out-of-pocket spending. Of the total number of households, 2.7% (3.8 million) were affected each year, either by catastrophic expenses that competed with the satisfaction of their basic needs, or by expenses that brought them below the level of poverty. The third imbalance was that of insufficient spending by state governments as compared with federal government spending. Thus, in 2000, the federal government contributed 84.8% of the total health system expenditure. The fourth imbalance was that of inequitable public expenditure. There was a profound inequity in the allocation of public health funding between the population with social insurance and those without it, with federal spending almost three times higher for the insured population. However, the allocation of federal resources to the states was also inequitable, in such a way that the Federal District (today, Mexico City) received up to 12 times more resources per capita than Guanajuato, while Baja California Sur, Colima and Aguascalientes received at least three times more resources than Puebla, Michoacán or the State of Mexico.

TABLE 6.1 Five financial imbalances motivating the SPSS, 2000 and 2014

NO.	IMBALANCE	NATURE OF THE IMBALANCE	2000	2014	% CHANGE 2000–2014[a]
1	Insufficient health spending (1)	National health spending as a % of GDP	5	6.3	26.0
2	Excessive out-of-pocket spending (2)	Out-of-pocket spending as a % of total health spending	55	43.2	−21.5
		Households with catastrophic health spending as a % of total households (2)	2.7	1.7	−37.0
3	Insufficient state government spending in health (1)	State government spending as a % of total public health spending	15.2	13.1	−13.8
4	Inequitable public health spending (1)	Per capita public health spending by social insurance institutions (pesos of 2014)	2283	5860	156.7
		Per capita public spending on the non-insured (pesos of 2014)	784	3641	364.4
		Ratio of per capita health spending between the insured and the non-insured	2.9	1.6	−43.4
		Ratio of federal per capita health spending in states with the most and the least spending	11.8	2.2	−81.4
5	High operational spending by the MoH (1)	Investment in infrastructure as a % of total health spending	3.7	1.7	−54.1
		Payroll spending as a % of total health spending	77	46	−40.3

[a]Constant pesos of 2014

Note: Italics denote changes unfavourable to correcting the disequilibria.

Sources: (1)Secretaría de Salud (2015d), (2)Knaul, Arreola Ornelas & Méndez Carniado (2016)

The fifth imbalance to overcome was that of high operating expenses and, correspondingly, the low expenditure on investment in health. In 2000, investment in health infrastructure was 4.0% of public spending, a worrying percentage above all due to the infrastructure deficit of a developing country undergoing an accelerated epidemiological transition. On the other hand, spending on human resources in health for the uninsured population among public providers corresponded to 77% of total public expenditure, an imbalance that hindered investment and innovation.

The five financial imbalances showed improvements in 2014, although not in all cases. That year national health expenditure as a percentage of GDP increased by 26.0%, to stand at 6.3%. Out-of-pocket spending showed a reduction of 21.5% while household catastrophic health expenditure, on the other hand, showed a reduction of 37%. Regarding the imbalance between public financing for the insured and the uninsured, the SPSS contributed to a notable improvement. The difference in public spending for the insured and the uninsured decreased from 3 times to 1.6 times higher. This happened as a result of greater increase in per capita spending for the uninsured than for the insured. The allocation of federal resources also became more equitable among the states, reducing maximum differences from 11 times to only twice the amount between the extreme states of Puebla and the Federal District.

There are, however, imbalances that did not improve and, on the contrary, worsened; such is the disparity between federal and state government contributions to the health services supporting the uninsured population as well as in investment expenditure more generally. State expenditure compared with federal expenditure showed a deterioration of 13.8% between 2000 and 2014, even though federal health financing was conditioned such that a proportional contribution was required by state governments. However, the situation was heterogeneous among the various states. Half showed decreases, particularly the states of Puebla, Morelos, Veracruz and Nuevo León. In contrast, states such as Oaxaca, Durango and the State of Mexico showed increases in their contributions. Investment in health infrastructure for the uninsured showed a reduction of 54.1%, despite the allocation of resources for investment available in the Budgetary Forecast Fund (FPP) of the SPSS trust, equivalent to 2% of the total SPSS fund. The expense of the payroll for human resources did show, nevertheless, progress towards what was expected; the reduction of its contribution by 40.3% freed up capital for spending on medicines and other health supplies.

6.3 Equity and efficiency impacts of SPSS

Seguro Popular made progress, leading to around 55 million Mexicans with financial protection for essential health services, while catastrophic health expenditures decreased by about a quarter (Knaul et al., 2012). However, universal health coverage was not attained, whether measured in terms of people covered, in access to essential interventions, in lowering of out-of-pocket expenditure or in strengthening pooled funding (see section 3.3.1). In spite of greater effective coverage for acute diseases and formal access to a set of cost-effective interventions, effective coverage for chronic care remained low. Diabetes is a case in point, with patients under control reaching only half that of the international standard. Out-of-pocket expenditures are still unduly high by upper middle-income country standards, at 41.5% of national health expenditure in 2014 (OECD, 2015). State contributions to pooled funding have remained below expectations, while contributions by individuals are far below what would be expected. Only 2% of the population that should have contributed to Seguro Popular actually do so, a loss representing 10% of Seguro Popular's funding (González Block et al., 2016).

Seguro Popular included a series of mechanisms that aimed to potentially achieve greater health system efficiency. An explicit package of services was defined to guarantee funding for priority interventions (CAUSES and the FPGC list). Funds were channelled to the newly established, specialized REPSS within state ministries of health. However, the lack of transparency and in some cases fund misallocation or even fraud at state level led to a reform in 2014 to re-establish REPSS as decentralized, autonomous units of state governments. Another change was the establishment of accounts with the Treasury of the Federation to avoid funds as far as possible being allocated to state treasuries. Funds were then channelled to REPSS based on the number of people registered in audited lists. Performance-based payment was encouraged either through performance agreements with public providers or through service contracts with private providers. However, no specific norms were established to foster the consolidation of performance-based payment and private providers are involved only as a last resource. Finally, there were initiatives for the use of innovative provider payment formulae, which included case-based payment for specialized care but can include other innovative mechanisms to target quality of care improvements.

Funding innovations made progress, with important limitations. High-cost interventions were gradually added, from an initial 49 in 2003 to 69 in 2018 (CNPSS, 2018b). Important interventions remain unfunded, such as the care for renal insufficiency and for cardiac infarction for patients over 60 – this last being the leading cause of death in Mexico. The normative procedure in place to add interventions to the basic package is limited to the analysis of interventions by the General Health Board, although it lacks a policy framework to prioritize pending interventions and to determine funding according to resource availability. The gradual levelling of benefits with respect to IMSS is thus in limbo.

During Seguro Popular expansion between 2003 and 2012, state governments enrolled mostly the easy-to-reach poor, non-contributory population to accelerate enrolment and to access additional federal funds. Equity was improved in so far as financial allocations and the improvement of infrastructure were concerned. As mentioned, millions of higher earners were enrolled for free, thereby not only failing to contribute to financing, but also weakening the focus on the poor; today up to 4.4 million rural poor remain outside Seguro Popular (González Block et al., 2018c). Free riding by the uninsured poor and the middle class was promoted by enabling registration when visiting the emergency room prior to major procedures.

Performance agreements signed by state Seguro Popular managers and public providers were pro-forma, focusing on general targets that were not tied to specific funding or to sanctions for non-compliance. Most of Seguro Popular funding and strategic focus were devoted to the purchase of inputs – drugs and medical personnel – rather than to the purchasing of services. This meant specialized state payers focused on tasks not much different from those covered by historical-based funding, although – importantly – greater capacity was given to identify funding flows for specific purchases. Furthermore, additional inputs made possible with greater Seguro Popular funding were administered in uncreative ways: new personnel were hired through temporary professional contracts of questionable legality, as doctors were deployed not as independent professionals but as subordinated workers. Yet they were denied the entitlements enjoyed by other doctors who had been contracted based on historical-based budgets and with whom they worked side by side. Facing protests, state and federal authorities proceeded to incorporate a large number of the recently hired health workers into standard, trade-unionized contracts whose funding was channelled along traditional funding routes, independently of REPSS. As for drugs, corruption scandals led to recentralized funding through a national purchasing mechanism.

6.4 **Demand-side funding by SPSS**

SPSS only partially achieved its aim of shifting funding from the supply side based on historical funding to the demand side based on performance-based payments. Out of the total funding mobilized by the System of Social Protection in Health, 48% was managed by national and state Seguro Popular managers and 52% was allocated through historical budgets tied to collective agreements (González Block et al., 2016). Only around 10% of Seguro Popular's high-specialty care providers were contracted from the private sector, while preference was given to public providers regardless of cost or quality. Only the state of Hidalgo implemented a contracting-out scheme to provide the essential primary care package of services through a private provider paid on a capitated basis estimated on the number of enrolled individuals in the community where the doctor team was practising. An evaluation suggests that this approach was cost-effective, although national authorities were reluctant to showcase it (Figueroa Lara & González Block, 2016). Case-based payment for specialized care of specific treatment pathways improved access and continuity of care as well as productivity, although fell short of improving quality. A case in point is breast cancer care, where case detection and treatment are paid separately, the latter receiving more pay for late-stage cancer cases and thus providing no incentives to liaise with primary care providers to ensure timely referrals (Lozano et al., 2013).

Strategic purchasing to maximize health requires the alignment of incentives across fund and health care management teams. Yet Seguro Popular fund managers remained in most cases wedded to public health providers and, as already stated, focused on non-strategic purchasing of inputs. Health service providers, for their part, lack decision-making autonomy to sell services and make rational use of resources. In fact, Seguro Popular is perceived as having contributed to a loss in hospital autonomy as out-of-pocket expenditure was abolished for most interventions, depriving hospitals of much-needed cash.

Furthermore, Seguro Popular in no way influenced hospital management capacity, as funds were only allocated to personnel in contact with patients and not for administrators. Corruption is a big problem at the state levels and spurred the centralization of purchasing of inputs, reducing further managerial responsibility.

Another challenge to the strategic management of funds by SPSS was the fact that a large part of the Seguro Popular population is transient, fluidly entering and exiting the formal labour market. Up to 38% of formal private sector workers covered by IMSS will lose their medical care rights due to exiting the formal sector at least once a year. Most would become potential Seguro Popular beneficiaries (Guerra et al., 2018). Yet Seguro Popular and IMSS do not speak to each other to ensure the continuity of financial protection, less so continuity of care. Clearly, efficient allocations will not be attained in Mexico through sequestering public funds within segmented, unresponsive institutions.

■ 6.5 **Portability and convergence**

The administration of president Felipe Calderón between 2006 and 2012 aimed to achieve universal coverage through the coordination of public federal institutions and state ministries of health following a strategy of portability and convergence. Compliance with the Millennium Development Goals, and in particular with the reduction of maternal mortality, were among the key motivators. Portability was defined as the capacity of all citizens to access public institutions regardless of the public payer behind them, while convergence aimed to create the mechanisms to enable portability.

The strategy aimed to address public hospital capacity imbalances, where some hospitals – particularly the new hospitals created by Seguro Popular – were operating under capacity, while others, especially at IMSS and ISSSTE, were saturated. IMSS hospitals operating at full occupancy often coexist with underused facilities. The strategy also aimed to contain overall costs, especially after the economic crisis of 2009. The federal government launched a service exchange agreement programme in 2011 to address this challenge through federal and state coordinating commissions and undertook capacity assessments based on patient guarantees and a catalogue of interventions and prices (see Box 6.1).

BOX 6.1 High-specialty exchange agreements

Authorities have promoted Collaboration and Coordination Agreements in the matter of Provision of Specialized Medical Services and Economic Compensation that allow payment for specific care across public hospitals regardless of their institution. A total of 715 clinical and surgical interventions, treatments, diagnostic tests and imaging studies are included in the agreements. However, there are no specific protocols to determine if external care is warranted according to health needs and service capacity, save for general waiting times (Secretaría de Salud, 2011). The effectiveness of agreements across institutions remains limited, lacking economic incentives to receive new cases given the low amounts paid or the lack of incentives to increase the productivity of the health team. According to IMSS, between 2012 and 2016 a total of 3658 patients per year on average were referred to other public institutions, while IMSS attended to 439 patients from other institutions (IMSS, 2017).

On the other hand, patients lack the power to choose treatment outside their institution when facing delays or other circumstances, so they do not promote the referral. Regardless of the normative regulation, patients frequently demand care from providers outside their institution or seek care outside their residency area, in response to perceptions of quality or due to mobility (González Block et al., 2011).

Even though the exchange agreements represent an important advance to address specific health problems, their management remains limited due to operational complications. In general, the care units lack economic incentives to receive new cases given the low amounts paid or the lack of incentives to increase the productivity of the health team. On the other hand, patients lack the power to choose their provider, so they do not promote the agreements. Regardless of the normative regulation, patients frequently demand care from providers outside their institution or seek care outside their residency area responding to perception of quality or due to mobility (González Block et al., 2011). These situations reflect a health system based on a segmented model with financial and coverage inequalities (Gómez Dantés et al., 2011).

Portability was encouraged through the development of various mechanisms for patient registration and information interchange. A national patient register was proposed but not implemented, and today only a mechanism exists to identify duplicated names registered across institutions. Electronic medical records (EMRs) were encouraged to enable the exchange of records as patients flowed across the system. EMRs were regulated through a national norm to specify standards and information interchange and efforts to implement EMRs were particularly strong within MoH facilities given their lag with respect to IMSS. Seguro Popular funded implementation projects mostly led by state authorities. In 2011, all IMSS hospitals and primary care facilities had EMRs, buy only 25% of MoH hospitals had them, and almost none were to be found among primary care facilities (González Block & López Santibañez, 2011).

Convergence of quality standards across institutions was promoted through clinical practice guidelines (CPGs), a health resources master plan, coordination for the acquisition of medicines and inputs, and common guidelines for training and human resource planning. Previous sections have developed some of these programmes (see sections 2.2 and 5.4.1). CPGs were elaborated by interinstitutional teams coordinated by the MoH, following common procedures and standards. Emphasis was given to writing and development of close to 700 CPGs, yet implementation lagged behind due to slow processes and few incentives to ensure application (Gutiérrez, González Block & Reyes, 2015).

The portability and convergence strategy was continued by the administration of Enrique Peña Nieto (2012–2018), although with less impetus. While state agreements for the exchange of patients were simplified and promoted, in 2015 only 11 agreements had been signed, with low levels of patient exchanges within signatory states. The low levels of implementation have been attributed in part to the lack of financial incentives. The catalogue of services established unit prices that are lower than costs within IMSS, while the lack of hospital autonomy and the difficulties to pay across public institutions remain important barriers (Health Research Institute, 2017).

6.6 **Persistence of segmentation**

President Enrique Peña Nieto was elected as a PRI candidate promising structural reforms that had not been enacted by the two previous opposition PAN administrations. Among the reforms undertaken were the introduction and strengthening of private investment throughout the energy economy and increasing competition in telecommunications. In education, teacher evaluation and transparent recruitment and promotion criteria were introduced, reducing the hold of trade unions. While it was expected that health policies would be reformed to introduce greater MoH oversight of social insurance institutions, Peña Nieto's presidency was in fact characterized by the continuity of previous policies. IMSS coverage was extended to specific groups defined by occupation, as was the case with secondary education students, and expanded to small businesses, incentivizing coverage of the latter by exempting them from paying contributions in the first years. IMSS coverage increased slightly over the period 2012–2018. In addition, improved administration and financial management led to the elimination of the operational deficit. However, the IMSS workers' pension fund deficit is increasing, which threatens to bankrupt IMSS within a few years.

The funding guidelines of SPSS and the administrative apparatus of Seguro Popular were reformed during the Peña Nieto administration to avert the financial mismanagement that became apparent in 2012, when fraud was denounced in a few states. Most of the funding was now retained by the federation in treasury accounts through which states could purchase drugs, while state ministries of health were directed to establish autonomous administrative units to handle registration and financial management. Specific limits and penalties were established to ensure timely financial allocation and to prevent fraud (González Block et al., 2018b).

6.7 **Future developments**

Federal officials and public policy-makers along most of the political spectrum together with non-government agencies developed a broad consensus between the late 1980s and the first decade of the new century on the challenges facing the consolidation of the National Health System, particularly those concerning the non-insured. The advent of President Andrés Manuel López Obrador leaves open the question of whether such a consensus will persist, particularly regarding the separation of functions of purchasing and provision.

6.7.1 *The current consensus*

The current consensus stresses the importance of integrating the different sources of public financing for health within a universal fund through the coordination of general taxes with social insurance contributions. Public health services should be freely available to all regardless of occupational employment or socioeconomic status. Less consensus exists with regards to collaboration with the private sector, with some proposals focusing almost entirely on creating a universal public system. The integration of a single fund with social insurance contributions and the various tax-based programmes has been discussed, yet never by Congress or at the highest levels of government. Indeed, the federal pact and the different sources of federal and state funding pose a particular challenge in this respect. The need to separate the functions of financial allocation and those of health services provision has also been proposed to achieve greater equity and efficiency in the management of public health resources (Auditoría Superior de la Federación, 2016; Grupo de trabajo de la Fundación Mexicana para la Salud, 2013; Murayama Rendón & Ruesga Benito, 2016; Narro Robles, Cordera Campos & Lomelí Venegas, 2006; 2010; Martínez Valle & Molano Ruíz, 2013). However, no broad consensus has been achieved, and indeed the administration of President López Obrador is moving in a different direction, towards the consolidation of funding and provision as well as strengthening the segmentation across social insurance and tax-based funding.

The importance of the decentralization of health services as an area of opportunity has also been discussed, recognizing the role that local authorities can play in responding to health needs, but also the need to increase their administrative capacity and probity. However, the administration of President López Obrador has tended to recentralize government in general, and health in particular. The aim is to establish INSABI as a centralized body similar to IMSS, with the capacity to enact vertical policies firmly under the control of the president and away from state governments, perceived as corrupt and inefficient.

Proposals also recognize the need to significantly reduce out-of-pocket expenses, improve the efficiency of public institutions and increase insured spending and investment. In addition, it has been stressed that there is a need to carry out reforms that allow the population to demand and receive health services where they find this most convenient and where the quality of care is guaranteed. While the administration of President López Obrador promised in the electoral campaign to integrate IMSS, IMSS Prospera and MoH health services, reforms actually moved in a different direction with the substitution of Seguro Popular by INSABI, thus perpetuating segmentation and reducing choice and demand-side incentives towards offering quality care.

These discussions about the challenges facing the Mexican health system have revealed the necessity of a new legal framework that directly addresses the specification of services to be financed with public funds, purchasing in the public and private spheres with criteria of efficiency and quality, and particularly, the establishment of a national agency to regulate health service provision (OECD, 2016).

In 2012, the Mexican Health Foundation (Funsalud) (Grupo de trabajo de la Fundación Mexicana para la Salud, 2013) identified challenges to finance the SPSS, since the expansion of interventions, as well as population coverage, depends on general taxes which are subject to the sway of the economy. Funsalud noted, in addition, the challenges facing FPGC's financial capacity and the impending deficit for 2025 if current funding is maintained. Funsalud thus raised the need for fiscal reform to increase the resources available, as well as measures to optimize the efficiency and quality of management and health services provision at state level.

Some study groups have agreed on the importance of the separation of functions between payers and providers, together with a stronger role for MoH health system governance (Martínez Valle & Molano Ruíz, 2013). The OECD analysed Mexico's health system in 2016 to identify future areas for development and reform. Four broad areas of recommendations were identified: 1) centring the health system on patients and people; 2) defining a universal package of benefits focused on primary care and prevention with continuity of care and pay-for-performance; 3) unifying financing across public institutions to improve efficiency and equity; and 4) health service performance monitoring focusing on quality and efficiency (OECD, 2016).

The role of the private health sector has not been fully addressed, although studies with sector leaders have identified a willingness to engage in public–private collaboration. The segmentation and subordination of the private sector by public policy has been recognized as a problem, particularly given the high level of uncoordinated private demand for services and the key role played by the pharmaceutical and medical device industries (González Block et al., 2018b). There is a broad consensus in the private sector on the importance of strengthening regulation and accreditation, both by government and by professional associations, as to ensure a level playing field for all actors and particularly to ensure uniform quality standards. Private providers have ample opportunities to focus on comprehensive primary health care and to develop information systems focusing on quality and efficiency. It is widely recognized that public–private collaboration is critical to attain the levels of investment required by the health system as a whole. Innovative private financing models have been envisioned in collaboration with social insurance institutions to complement health service coverage. It has also been recognized that integrating the private sector within the NHS requires it to open itself to areas of collaboration through explicit regulations as well as developing its own leadership capacity.

Analyses of the challenges posed by IMSS's corporatist governance structure identified broad issues that need short-term resolution (González Block, 2018). Among the most challenging are recognizing the lack of congruence between social insurance coverage and the labour market, with the informal sector as the main player and, above all, a rapid and continuous turnover of workers across the formal and informal labour markets. This reality strengthens the recommendation of moving towards the separation of functions, not only to improve efficiency, but to ensure continuity of care in a context of the chronic diseases now prevalent in the country. However, separation of functions may not be enough to encourage efficiency, and there remains a need to focus on competition between financial managers and between providers.

A major pending issue is the technical bankruptcy of IMSS, where unfunded entitlements threaten to absorb an increasing amount of operational income. Funding entitlements out of current income will be untenable soon, as it is projected that by 2030 up to 63% of income would be absorbed by the pension fund (González Block, 2018). Addressing this situation may require additional taxation or debt, something that could provoke a political crisis. The government could also consider increasing IMSS workers' productivity and income through pay-for-performance, where additional income is directed to pay for entitlements.

The magnitude of changes required within IMSS and across the health system calls for an overhaul of institutional and health system governance, introducing professional managers and boards in lieu of corporative appointees from worker and employer unions. Furthermore, health service providers should be given greater autonomy to assume risk and to introduce incentives towards efficiency and quality.

■ **6.7.2** *The emerging consensus*

The current health policy aims to strengthen the public health system along its segmented architecture and on the basis of the right to health protection, rather than a universal right to health as enshrined in the Treaty of Economic, Cultural and Social Rights, recognized by the Constitution. The policy objectives stated in the Sectoral Health Plan 2019–2024 aim to achieve universal coverage through strengthening the efficiency of government health providers. Free and accessible services from the first level of care all the way up to specialized care are expected to reduce inequalities in health and to bring chronic diseases to a halt, as well as to significantly reduce out-of-pocket expenditure (Secretaría de Salud, Programa Sectorial de Salud 2019–2024).

As with other areas of government, the principles of the current administration's health policy platform stress first and foremost good governance with ethical commitments towards efficiency, transparency and probity. Universalization of coverage would be pursued to guarantee equality of access, health service quality and financial equity. Importantly, the poor and those excluded from coverage would be prioritized to guarantee that all Mexicans are covered by "equivalent health services". The social determinants of health would be addressed together with care targeting vulnerable groups to ensure integral care for specific needs. Social and citizen participation and collaboration will be pursued with an intersectoral approach for policy formulation and programme implementation. Evaluation, transparency and accountability across the health system will target its adequate operation and the fight against corruption. Finally, financial solidarity will be pursued through the equitable contribution of every person's income.

The points of action enshrined by the current government include the transformation of the health system towards primary health care based on integrated care networks. The proposal would prioritize community health care units and public health initiatives with an intersectoral approach involving industry. The public health system would be strengthened through coordinated objectives and collaboration of federal and state providers, promoting the stewardship of the federal government and citizen surveillance. Social control and participation would be pursued through prioritizing humane and proficient care supported by participation in informed dialogue.

Combating corruption and improving resource administration are initiatives to be pursued through public bidding and a national registry of providers. A pharmaceutical and health inputs policy will be developed to favour national producers in both the public and private sectors while prescription and use of medications will be improved through technology and pharmacovigilance.

At least 1% of GDP will be allocated in additional public funding for public providers. Quality of care will be pursued through integrating additional resources and improvements to organizations that place the patient and the community at their centre. Emergency care will be strengthened to respond to the most common incidents and natural disasters, while WHO's recommended "Health in all policies" will be implemented. Health research will focus on the most representative diseases, of which the platform highlights degenerative and muscular-skeletal diseases, chronic renal insufficiency, maternal and child nutrition, environmental health and climate change. Finally, health information and evaluation systems will be strengthened with a focus on citizens and governmental evaluators.

This broad and ambitious platform faces the challenge of ensuring the financing required as well as the efficiency in its administration. Past policies have proven that segmentation is a major barrier for efficiency, while the federal nature of government in Mexico requires effective coordination and incentives for collaboration. Dismantling the separation of financing and provision within the MoH aims to ensure integrated care; however, relying on historical funding based on the supply side may prove a major hurdle to attain efficiency.

7

Assessment of the health system

■ Chapter summary

- Health policy in Mexico since 2000, and up until 2018 at least, has been characterized by the pursuit of universal health coverage following the 1983 Decree of the Right to Health Protection.
- Out-of-pocket spending decreased slightly, with important reductions in catastrophic expenditure thanks to Seguro Popular and possibly also to the role of generic medicines and low-cost private consultations.
- While Seguro Popular provided an explicit package of benefits, critical high-specialty interventions are still not covered for the non-insured.
- The Mexican health system is faced with shortages and imbalances in health resources affecting nurses, medical specialists and personnel with innovative competencies to address health promotion and prevention.
- Per capita public health spending decreased for the first time in decades as a result of small but significant reductions in the funding for the non-insured.
- The segmented governance of the health system is perhaps the biggest obstacle to a universal health system, given that social insurance institutions cannot be regulated by the MoH.

- This situation hinders the development of a stronger regulatory authority capable of addressing access barriers and quality of care.
- The objective to establish a universal national health system fell short of expectations during the Peña Nieto administration, with health policy maintaining the segmentation of the health system.
- The administration of President Andrés Manuel López Obrador has promised to integrate the health system and end segmentation during its tenure from 2018 to 2024.

7.1 **Health system governance**

7.1.1 *Transparency and accountability*

The Mexican government and particularly the health system have striven to become more transparent and accountable in the face of corruption and clientelism. The federal government now requires each service facility to implement procedures to comply with the National Law of Access to Public Information, whereby any citizen can request information and receive an answer within a specified period as regulated by the National Institute for Transparency and Access to Public Information and Data Protection (INAI). The Social Insurance Law was reformed in the early 2000s to ensure financial accountability in the face of deficits and mismanagement, requiring an annual audit by a private firm and the publication of a report to Congress and the federal executive. However, the report is produced by the IMSS General Directorate and the Directorate for Finances, and not by the controlling body, the technical council, which is the authority accountable to Congress according to the Social Insurance Law. Reporting by IMSS is characterized by service provision statistics and not service demand and benefits provided to its affiliates, although isolated efforts are made to implement quality of care surveys.

The MoH increased transparency and accountability through the explicit packages of benefits and financial architecture of Seguro Popular. The list of benefits was regularly updated and published, and the compliance with the list of benefits was continuously assessed at the patient and facility level. Financial contributions and terms were clearly established at the federal and state level, with explicit reporting mechanisms aiming to ensure timely disbursement. Governing boards were established at state level to ensure that the decentralized funding management agents, the REPSS, performed according to expectations. The CNPSS was also obliged to provide an annual report on its finances and coverage to Congress and the federal executive. With the substitution of Seguro Popular by INSABI all these mechanisms have been abolished and no alternative mechanisms have been implemented. Even when Seguro Popular was in place, the population was still largely disenfranchised from health institutions and services, as it lacks a Patient's Charter, information systems and mechanisms to empower public demand of services (see section 2.6).

◼ **7.1.2** *Public participation*

The health system of Mexico is characterized by vertical public institutions governed through corporatist boards or through political appointees, with little if any horizontal participation by citizens, patients or consumers. Governing councils of autonomous hospitals and of REPSS at state level excluded the participation of citizen representatives. The National Health Council through which health sector policy is formulated includes only the participation of public and social insurance health institution decision-makers and excludes the participation of private sector providers and of civil society organizations (see section 2.5). The General Health Council, charged with accreditation and the inclusion of medical inputs within institutional lists, does not include the participation of patient organizations but does include the participation of NGOs, mostly professional organizations.

Given the structure of representation in place, patients are limited in their capacity to influence treatment decisions, with only informed consent being made available prior to interventions. Neither citizens nor patients can influence purchasing decisions by political or administrative means and are left only with recourse to out-of-pocket purchasing when medicines are not dispensed, or when waiting times for treatment are unduly prolonged. The only mechanism available to support patients voicing complaints – the National or State Commissions for Medical Arbitration – are limited to medical complaints and have no binding authority.

■ **7.1.3** *Health system performance monitoring and research*

Social policy and programme evaluation in Mexico are regulated through the General Social Development Law that established the National Council for the Evaluation of Social Development Policy (CONEVAL). CONEVAL designs, coordinates and executes studies and is responsible for the measurement of poverty indicators and for the evaluation of the attainment of social policy objectives across ministries and institutions. CONEVAL has pioneered mandatory programme evaluation worldwide and for health policy, which has been particularly important in measuring financial protection gaps (Oxman et al., 2010). Among its findings, CONEVAL reported that the reduction of financial protection gaps in health has been particularly successful thanks to Seguro Popular, showing the fastest such reduction across social policy indicators in the past 10 years (CONEVAL, 2018).

The MoH regulates and funds health policy and programme evaluation in line with CONEVAL through the General Directorate for Performance Evaluation (DGED). DGED focuses on strengthening the NHS through sector evaluations and diagnostics undertaken internally and extramurally and focusing mostly on MoH and state health institutions.

Health research is primarily funded through federal resources channelled into the Sectoral Fund for Basic Research and the Sectoral Fund for Research in Health and Social Security (FOSISS). Federal and state funds were until 2018 also pooled through the Mixed Funds, all administered by CONACYT (Martínez Martínez et al., 2012). In 2010, total research spending on health amounted to 1.1% of the national public health budget, and funding did not significantly increase up until 2018. FOSISS was funded by equal contributions by the MoH, IMSS and ISSSTE, and pools funds through a national yearly competition. CONACYT also plays a key role for health research through funding the National Researchers System, a member-based, performance-related grants system with 2800 members working in medicine and the health sciences (Rodríguez, 2016). The MoH has the strongest presence in basic, clinical and health systems research, followed by IMSS. MoH research infrastructure is housed in 13 National Institutes of Health in Mexico City and Cuernavaca, while IMSS has a national coordination centre and local centres in some of its high-specialty hospitals and regional units across the country. The MoH and IMSS have their own internationally indexed health research journals. The journal Salud Pública de México has chronicled policy and programme development and impact mostly within the MoH for the past 50 years, while the Archives of Biomedical Research edited by IMSS focuses on biomedical and clinical research.

■ **7.1.4** *Health information systems*

Mexico's health information system faces the challenge of institutional segmentation and barriers to effective coordination as well as the fragmentation and poor regulation of the private sector. The main issues are the lack of comparable information on available resources, the lack of focus on quality of care and cost indicators, and health-need information gaps, particularly in the case of the national cancer registry. Due to the distinct structures of the information subsystems, including the surveys and the different data sets, as well as the problem of sub-diagnoses of diseases, national data on disease incidence and prevalence are still incomplete. The quality of health information has been addressed through training and normative coordination, leading to WHO-certified quality levels in areas such as infant and maternal deaths.

■ 7.2 **Accessibility**

Mexico's health system imposes many health service access barriers in spite of extensive policies to ensure coverage (see section 3.3.1). Up to 38% of IMSS beneficiaries lose their entitlements per year due to moving out of the private sector labour market, mostly when taking up jobs in the informal sector (Guerra et al., 2018). Even chronic disease patients are exposed to this barrier, as suggested by the fact that 32% of IMSS beneficiaries being treated for diabetes lose access to IMSS in a period of 3 years (Doubova et al., 2018). Furthermore, as the uninsured gain access to IMSS, they are forced to seek care with IMSS providers. Social insurance institutions lack capacity to provide services to all their enrollees, mostly due to resource shortages. Hence up to 35% of social insurance beneficiary outpatient consultations and 17% of inpatient services are provided by the private sector. Similar access barriers are presented by MoH providers catering to the uninsured, with 33% being forced to use private outpatient services and 15% in the case of inpatient services (González Block et al., 2018b). The private sector has thus developed to relieve public sector access barriers through low-cost services.

There is evidence of inequity in the use of health services, since households with fewer resources, less education and located in areas of high marginalization have a higher probability of not using outpatient services when they need them, compared with the population with greater resources, better education and who reside in urban areas. Supply side barriers, such as the absence of service providers close to home or having to pay for services, are the main causes of inequality and are cited by those who choose not to seek care, at a rate 2.5 times higher among households in the lower income quintile compared with those in the highest quintile (Bautista Arredondo et al., 2014).

The distribution of health resources among states is also uneven, and is concentrated on the main cities of the country, especially the capital. The shortage of personnel and technology in rural areas is notable. Section 7.4 addresses inequity issues in outcomes that are closely related to inequity in access to services.

Overall, while the Mexican health system provides support to most of the population for most of their health needs, the experience of users has clear opportunities for improvement. While no single study or system is in place to thoroughly inform about the perception of users with regard to specific services and situations, the highly fragmented patient care pathways and lack of coordination across public and private institutions described in sections 5.2 and 5.3 suggests that dissatisfaction is common across all socioeconomic groups and that persons living with chronic diseases are particularly affected. Effective coverage studies have suggested that institutions are not being managed with the patients clearly in mind.

A study on effective coverage of breast cancer suggests that only 1.2% of women with confirmed diagnoses enter treatment on time according to international guidelines (Uscanga et al., 2014). This must be accompanied by delays in care associated with negative experiences, although again, these should be studied in detail. The lack of empowerment by users vis-à-vis payers and providers, the lack of information systems oriented to users and the predominance of top-down interest representation mechanisms leave little option to users but to seek care with private providers.

A study of people with diabetes and/or hypertension in urban areas of Mexico found that up to 39% sought care in a period of 1 year with both social insurance and private providers, while 44.6% were loyal to their public provider and 16.3% chose to see only a private doctor (Health Research Institute, 2017). The daily experience with services is therefore one of seeking care with medical providers in nearby locations providing fast, low-cost services whose focus may be more on symptomatic care rather than on disease control, and demanding services with institutional providers when costlier care or medicines are required.

7.3 **Financial protection**

SPSS and its operating arm, the Seguro Popular, implemented the right to health protection aiming to universalize free access to a broad package of benefits and reduce catastrophic health expenditure. The implementation of SPSS was associated with the reduction of catastrophic and impoverishing health spending, which affected 10.0% of households in 2000 and showed a marked reduction to 3.3% in 2012 (Knaul et al., 2012). However, other factors may also have contributed to this reduction, such as the expansion of low-cost medical care based on generic drugs and the care of physicians adjacent to pharmacies, as suggested by the fact that the slope of the curve in the reduction of excessive expenditure is similar to that across those insured by Seguro Popular and the non-insured (Figure 7.1). However, in 2018 up to 14.5% of Mexicans did not have financial protection in health, while access barriers to pre-paid services persist, keeping out-of-pocket spending at levels well above other upper middle-income countries (Peña Nieto, 2017).

FIG. 7.1 Proportion (%) of households reporting catastrophic and impoverishing health expenditures, 1992–2012

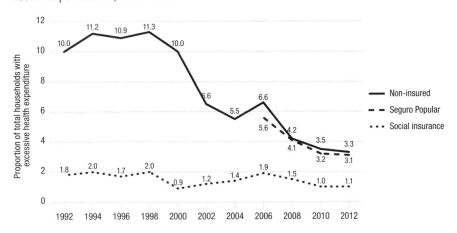

Source: Modified from Knaul et al. (2012)

Social protection in health through Seguro Popular prioritized the poorest populations, providing 87.3% of protection for those in the income quintile 1 – the poorest – in 2016. In contrast, social insurance institutions contributed 75.5% of the financial protection for the population in the fifth quintile of income (authors' calculation based on ENSANUT 2016). Seguro Popular contributed to equalizing the proportion of the population without health insurance coverage across income groups from 2000 to 2012, with a somewhat increased gap observed for 2016. Indeed, when comparing the percentage of people without financial protection across the two extreme income groups, the ratio went from 0.47 in 2000 (nearly twice as many of the poorest without insurance) to 0.65 in 2006 and to 0.99 in 2012 (Gutiérrez et al., 2016). For 2016, this ratio lowered to 0.89, suggesting a slight increase in financial protection inequity (INEGI, 2016a). The package of services protected for the non-insured through Seguro Popular is more limited, as discussed in section 2.3.1, and has not increased significantly since its roll-out in 2004.

The ratio of the proportion of excessive spending among the extreme income quintiles was also reduced, passing from 2.6 in 2004 to 1.8 in 2014 (Gutiérrez et al., 2016; Knaul, Arreola Ornelas & Méndez Carniado, 2016). However, households in income quintile 1 spend on average 303 Mexican pesos per year in outpatient medical care, versus 1552 pesos in quintile 5 (authors' processing of ENSANUT 2012). Differences in expenditure are similar to differences in the average total household income across extreme quintiles, suggesting that the impact of out-of-pocket expenditure is greater for the poorest households and, therefore, inequitable.

The Healthcare Access and Quality (HAQ) Index, which ranges from 0 (worst performance) to 100 (best performance), combines information on avoidable mortality with access to services provided by the health system. According to the most recent data, in 2016 Mexico reached a level of 66.3, higher than Brazil (63.8) but the lowest among OECD countries (IHME, 2018) (Figure 7.2).

At the subnational level, the distribution of the HAQ Index is unequal, with the Mexican states with greater poverty, such as Chiapas (HAQ=55.8), Oaxaca (HAQ=59.5) and Guerrero (HAQ=60.0) to the south, being those with less access to quality health care. In contrast, the northern states with greater wealth, such as Nuevo León (HAQ=72.8), Mexico City (HAQ=72.4), Tamaulipas (HAQ=72.3) and Sinaloa (HAQ=71.6), have greater access and quality (Figure 7.3).

FIG. 7.2 Healthcare Access and Quality (HAQ) Index, Mexico and selected countries, 2016

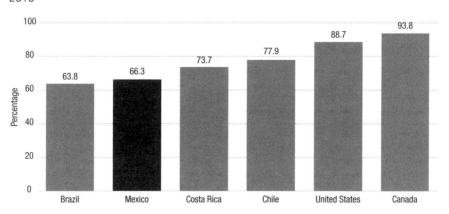

Source: Authors, based on IHME (2018) data

FIG. 7.3 Healthcare Access and Quality (HAQ) Index, Mexico, by state, 2016

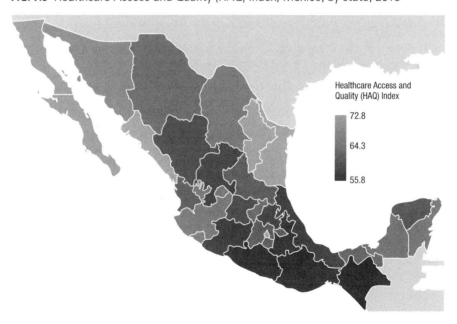

Source: Authors, based on IHME (2018) data

■ 7.4 **Health care quality**

Quality of care in Mexico is difficult to assess in comparison to other countries, given the differences in access barriers. The hospital admission rate due to uncontrolled diabetes in Mexico, for example, is below the average for OECD countries (66.3 vs 137.2 cases per 10 000 inhabitants), yet diabetes represents the primary cause of mortality in Mexico.

Mortality due to acute myocardial infarction (AMI) suggests that quality of care is widely differentiated across providers. Between 1998 and 2015, deaths increased by 87.4%, mostly as a result of the epidemiological transition. AMI mortality 30 days after diagnosis in Mexico is reported at an alarming rate of 28 per 100 discharges, which is close to four times higher than the OECD average of close to 7 per 100 discharges (Azpiri, 2016). However, among private hospitals larger than 100 beds, AMI mortality was measured at 3.1 cases per 100 discharges, below the OECD average. While AMI mortality among social insurance institutions doubles to 6.5 per 100 discharges, Azpiri infers that much higher mortality must be occurring within hospitals that serve the population without social insurance or in smaller private hospitals – as high as 59% – so as to explain the national rate of 28 per 100 discharges. This observation acquires additional weight when noting that the largest private hospitals concentrate 70% of the haemodynamic equipment in Mexico, while Seguro Popular did not cover the financing of AMI treatments for patients over 60 years of age.

The quality of care for women's health has shown a mixed evolution. The proportion of pregnant women who received their first prenatal consultation in the first trimester of pregnancy corresponded to 84.3% in 2012 (Gutiérrez et al., 2012). In the case of caesarean births, there has been, however, an upward trend from 2000, from 29.9% of total births to 45.2% in 2012, a challenge given the recommendation of international organizations not to exceed 15% of caesarean births of total births (García Alonso, 2015). Furthermore, births among adolescent women in Mexico, at 66.2 per 1000 in 2016, is over five times the OECD rate and one third higher than in Chile (OECD, 2018e).

In the case of the complete supply of medical prescriptions across public institutions, this ranged from 64% to 86% of total prescriptions in 2012, which is below what is desirable and which affects out-of-pocket expense (Gutiérrez et al., 2012). This deficit responds not only to deficiencies in planning, but also to the lack of incentives to ensure patient satisfaction given low-patient empowerment and to the problem of dissatisfaction among private, low-cost service providers.

7.5 **Health system outcomes**

7.5.1 *Population health*

Life expectancy in Mexico is above countries such as Brazil, Latvia, the Russian Federation and South Africa; but far below the 31 OECD countries led by Japan, Switzerland, Spain and Italy that reach a life expectancy of between 82.6 to 83.9 (OECD, 2018d). Life expectancy has increased more slowly in Mexico than in the rest of the OECD, thus increasing the relative gap between these countries (OECD, 2017a). Infant mortality has shown important improvements, with 12.1 deaths per 1000 live births in 2016 (World Bank, 2018). However, this figure is greater than all of the OECD countries but lower than the rate reported for Brazil, Colombia, Indonesia, South Africa and India.

7.5.2 *Equity of outcomes*

The health and life expectancy of the Mexican population are still highly influenced by differences in social circumstances, mainly in terms of education and income. Infant mortality rate (IMR) differences persist across states and municipalities, mostly related to their contrasting socioeconomic development. While the richest locality, the mayoralty of Benito Juárez in Mexico City, has an IMR of 3 per 1000 liveborn, the municipality of Cochoapa el Grande in Guerrero – among the poorest in the country – has an IMR of 61. The two most contrasting states in the country have IMRs of 13 in Mexico City, and 24 in Guerrero (CONAPO, 2005). These factors largely determine the type of health subsystem that people can access, particularly in the case of formal workers with access to social insurance. Healthy lifestyles also reveal great challenges in terms of the availability and consumption of healthy foods, physical activity, exposure to tobacco, alcohol, and drugs, and sexual and reproductive health factors, among others.

Indicators such as the Human Development Index, the Marginalization Index, the Multidimensional Measurement of Poverty (CONEVAL, 2016), and the measurement of the burden of disease in Mexico (Gómez Dantés, 2016), have been consistent in identifying regions or states that can be classified as vulnerable. Such is the case for the states of Chiapas, Guerrero, Oaxaca, Veracruz and Puebla, all of which are located immediately south of the State of Mexico. ENSANUT 2016 revealed challenges related to unfavourable indicators throughout the southern region (which adds the states of Campeche, Tlaxcala, Quintana Roo, Tabasco and Yucatán to the previous list). This region observed the highest prevalence of diabetes mellitus in adults 20 years and older in the country (10.2%) and the highest prevalence of overweight in adolescents (28.5%). Paradoxically, the southern region also observed the highest proportion of people aged 20 to 59 who perceived themselves as physically active (72.9%) and considered their diet healthy (64.0%).

Despite the inequality of out-of-pocket health expenditures and access to outpatient services, public health programmes have been able to increase effective coverage to preventive interventions, to the extent that the population in the lowest income quintile reports more access to certain interventions compared with the population in the highest quintile. Thus, the relative gap of access is progressive to mammograms, with a ratio of 2.5 between the lowest and highest quintile, and 1.8 for human papillomavirus vaccine. In the case of prenatal care, progressivity is lower, with a relative gap of 1.3, and in the case of early detection of cervical cancer it is 1.2. Access to care is indistinct at the socioeconomic level for interventions such as child delivery in hospitals and vaccination for measles, BCG and DPT (diphtheria, pertussis and tetanus). In contrast, care for diarrhoeal diseases and administration of the influenza vaccine is regressive (Gutiérrez et al., 2016).

Maternal mortality has shown important reductions, although this indicator failed to reach the levels set by the Millennium Development Goals. Furthermore, greater progress was made in better-off states and municipalities, leading to an increase in inequity with respect to this indicator. While in 2010 the relative gap across states considered best and worst according to the Human Development Index was 1.6, this indicator increased to reach 1.9 in 2012, and was 2.8 in 2014 (Freyermuth, Luna & Muños, 2014).

Progress in public health indicators is associated to increases in life expectancy in some poor states, such as Chiapas, Oaxaca and Puebla, with an increase of between 1.1 and 1.8 years between 2000 and 2013. Such increases are more notable given that nine states actually decreased their life expectancy during that period, most notably Colima, with 1.6 years lost, mostly due to violent deaths (Gómez Dantés et al., 2016).

7.6 **Health system efficiency**

The relationship between per capita health expenditure and life expectancy suggests that the Mexican health system is inefficient, in comparison with other countries. While Costa Rica and Chile spend similar amounts as Mexico on health per capita, their life expectancies are close to 5 years higher. Furthermore, increases in per capita health expenditure are associated with greater increases in life expectancy than in Mexico (Figure 7.4).

FIG. 7.4 Expenditure on health and life expectancy at birth (years), Mexico and selected OECD countries, 2000–2015

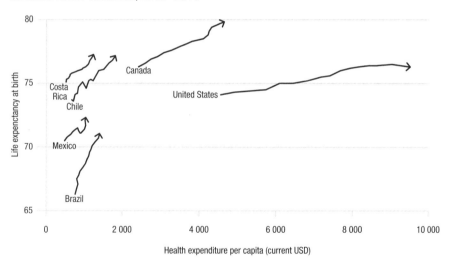

Source: OECD (2017b)

7.6.1 *Allocative efficiency*

Allocative efficiency is low given the fragmentation of the Mexican health system. As shown in Figures 3.6 and 3.7, financing flows are complex, since the money collected by the government is directed to different funds (social insurance, SPSS, state governments), with different allocation rules. Providers that have to seek different sources of funding must perform varied and complex planning exercises to achieve the allocation of expenditure. Providers for the non-insured have to access FASSA budget branches 12 (Health) and 19 (Seguro Popular, now INSABI), among the most important. FASSA is allocated directly to state governments and is mainly used to pay payroll for people who carry out activities for different programmes (CONEVAL, 2018). Branch 12, on the other hand, is intended to fund both administration and health care at the federal and state level, and funds health programmes under strict allocation rules. Financial management complexity is partly responsible for an overly high percentage of public health funding spent on administration and governance, with 4.8%, as against 2.9% the 2016 OECD average (OECD, 2018b).

■ 7.6.2 *Technical efficiency*

As seen in Chapter 4, the Mexican health system has insufficient human, infrastructure and technology resources to cover the population's demand for services, which undermines the technical impact of the resources that are allocated to health care.

A key organizational challenge affecting the efficiency of the Mexican health system is the diffuse boundary in the labour market between formal private sector employees and those in the informal sector. As mentioned in section 7.2, when discussing access barriers, every year 38% of employees covered by IMSS lose their formal employment, with more than half moving over to the informal sector or as independent workers without health benefits (Guerra et al., 2018). Labour mobility affects a larger proportion of the population when measured over a longer period of time than 1 year (Doubova et al., 2018). Such a frequent loss of coverage by IMSS challenges registration by Seguro Popular, as well as financial allocation and continuity of care. Indeed, a study of a cohort of IMSS patients with diabetes followed up during a 3-year period suggested that 32% lost medical coverage, which significantly reduced (by 43%) the likelihood that these patients received at least half of the recommended preventive measures. Patients who lost their IMSS coverage were also 19% less likely to control their diabetes, as measured by the indicator HbA1c at levels below 7% (Doubova et al., 2018).

Another organizational challenge is the efficient utilization of high-specialty health infrastructure, particularly tertiary care hospitals. Patients often have to travel long distances or wait longer to receive care within their own institution, when a high-specialty facility belonging to another institution may be nearby or may have greater availability. A recent study suggested that for up to 50% of adults in urban areas, the nearest hospital to them is not included in their insurance scheme, thus, leading them to travel longer distances to reach their designated facility (Health Research Institute, 2017).

A further organizational challenge is the fact that IMSS medical and allied personnel form part of the second largest trade union in Latin America, defending salaries and benefits higher than the average public or private sector employees. Unit costs at IMSS are up to three times those of state and federal government health services and the IMSS employee pension fund is bankrupt, with pensions absorbing an increasing proportion of institutional income and competing with operational and investment needs, yet still far insufficient to meet future needs (González Block, 2018) (see section 3.3). Vertical integration and lack of provider choice have led to a high degree of beneficiary dissatisfaction, contributing to the high level of out-of-pocket health expenditure to access private facilities across social strata.

8

Conclusions

Mexico has a large, highly diverse and ageing population settled in a complex landscape, mostly urbanized but also present in difficult-to-access rural areas. Economic inequality and poverty still affect ample sectors of the population, while chronic diseases constitute the prevalent health problem, deepening inequalities in health conditions and access to quality health services. While life expectancy has dramatically increased in the past decades, further gains are slow and disparities with respect to OECD countries are increasing. Health conditions vary widely across socioeconomic groups, with malnutrition a problem among the very poor.

Mexico's health system has evolved from centralized public health campaigns and a decentralized, mandatory private sector-led accident insurance system developed from the beginning of the 20th century towards a corporatist, authoritarian framework in the 1940s, aiming to control the social question through segmented, vertically structured, social insurance and social assistance institutions addressing industrialization and social differentiation. While the Constitution was amended in the 1980s to enshrine the right to health protection, this right was differentiated within the same Constitution according to the laws governing social insurance institutions and the MoH. This differentiated right enabled the development of the National Health System as a set of coordination committees across public institutions. However, segmentation persists as a major barrier to contend with new health care needs and demands, and is restricting public investment and expenditure, while instigating health service dissatisfaction and demand of a largely unregulated and uncoordinated private sector. Increased public spending has failed to substantially reduce out-of-pocket expenditures, although catastrophic expenditures have been significantly reduced. Out-of-pocket expenditures are at levels well beyond what is observed in more responsive health systems at similar or even lower levels of development.

Institutional segmentation restricts the regulatory reach of the MoH, which cannot legally enforce standards within social insurance institutions and is limited to their voluntary coordination. Yet social insurance institutions are highly centralized and are governed through corporatist arrangements focusing on the balancing of trade-unionized labour and employer interests, although the vast majority of beneficiaries are not trade unionized. IMSS has legitimated its privileged position through the provision of social assistance services funded by the federation based on a separate, far inferior infrastructure, thus further segmenting its relationship with the MoH.

The MoH was strengthened in the 2000s with the establishment of SPSS and Seguro Popular to increase funding and quality of care for the non-insured. While financial equity gaps were reduced and catastrophic expenditure curbed, SPSS did not address segmentation. However, greater parity in per capita expenditure across institutions as well as financial management innovations strengthened MoH leadership and made integration more feasible.

Integration seems the most promising option to follow, especially given that the labour market has remained highly unstable, with a large crossover between the formal labour market and the larger informal sector. Such crossover implies high levels of rotation of coverage between IMSS and Seguro Popular and, ultimately, the operation of two public institutions catering to the same population through different financial flows and infrastructures. Yet labour rotation is associated with a loss in quality of care, as patients are forced to change health care providers. Segmentation is associated with poor regulation in the health system as a whole, further bolstering poor quality, dissatisfaction and high out-of-pocket expenditures. The conjunction of corporatist centralism within social insurance and decentralized federalism in public health and social assistance has proven to be a major obstacle to health reform. This scenario hinders health promotion and the early detection and control of chronic diseases, ultimately affecting health expenditure, productivity and well-being.

Evidence suggests that the situation of the Mexican health system is characterized by inequity, segmentation and low levels of empowerment and satisfaction, which reflect its authoritarian corporatist structure. While many health systems in Latin America also shared a corporatist structure, health reforms in the majority have led to the development of more effective, unified and competitive health systems, with much lower levels of out-of-pocket expenditure and greater state role in their regulation (González Block & Martínez, 2015).

Mexico's health system is characterized by corporatism, similar to the corporatism of the health systems of Italy, Spain and Greece prior to the introduction of universal national health systems in the first two, and of a major reform in Greece to integrate the health system. Italy and Spain shed their corporatist health system structures in the 1970s and 1980s, towards universal, tax-funded and highly decentralized health systems (Ferré et al., 2014; García et al., 2010). Greece, on the other hand, established from 2011 provider choice across institutions that were previously exclusively for the benefit of specific occupational groups while also offering choice with private providers (Economou et al 2017). The Mexican health system thus shows almost point-by-point the traits found by Economou (2010) in the Greek health system prior to its reform, suggesting the influence of the following corporativist themes:

- High degree of centralization in decision-making and administrative processes, in spite of formal delegating to states responsibility for services for the non-insured.
- Ineffective managerial structures, governed by corporatist or local interests far removed from a health mandate and leading to separate infrastructures which cater, nonetheless, to a single population.
- Lack of system-wide health information management systems, with weak coordination of indicators and low levels of information sharing. This situation may change with the current integration into a single information platform, the National Basic Health Information System (SINBA), yet the lack of incentives towards a unified system may hinder progress.
- Lack of universal regulation, planning and coordination, driven through voluntary participation by social insurance and private sector institutions, a situation that weakens interest in developing more effective means of coordination.

- Unequal and inefficient allocation of human and economic resources still based on historical and political criteria in spite of efforts to increase funding for the non-insured. Regional disparities persist and are still glaring in health care outcomes.
- Inefficient resource allocation due to an absence of pooling of health resources, a lack of coordination among a limited number of public payers, an absence of adequate financial management and accounting systems, and a lack of financial monitoring processes.
- Fragmentation of coverage, with an uncoordinated private sector responding to the lack of satisfaction and capacity in the public sector and an absence of a referral system based on primary care. While interstate patient flows have been improved among the non-insured, labour rotation is high across the formal and informal sectors, erecting artificial barriers to health service access and leading to low levels of continuity of care.
- Inequalities in access to services derived from differences in financial protection coverage, high out-of-pocket payments and uneven urban–rural distribution of human resources and health infrastructure.
- Underdevelopment of regulation and policy coordination, including needs assessment and priority-setting mechanisms, which persist as official, top-down directives without ensuring wide social consensus.
- Regressive funding mechanisms due to the existence of high private spending; widespread tax evasion through the informal market.
- Predominance of salary-based payment systems among public providers and a limited range of fee-for-service or case-based payment mechanisms for selected interventions funded by Seguro Popular, resulting in the absence of incentives to improve efficiency and quality.

Our analysis suggests that a constitutional reform is required to establish a universal right to health dissociated from the underlying, segregationist legal framework behind social insurance institutions, the MoH and the private sector. Such a reform should place social insurance funding and health infrastructure on the same basis of federal- and state-controlled MoH funding and infrastructure. On this basis, public funding and providers should be able to improve their supply and, ultimately, identify the appropriate role for private providers.

A universal right to health would support the transformation of public institutions into more efficient and responsive entities, retaining their contributory financial architectures while separating functions for financial management, provision and regulation. The definition of a national, costed health package would be required, together with a fund to enable the gradual equalization of benefits. IMSS and MoH health facilities could be given administrative autonomy to offer services to local populations according to demand. Families would also be given the choice of being covered by IMSS or any other social insurance institution – or even by a new cadre of private financial managers established through a statutory law.

Integration implies transforming the current corporatist governance of IMSS into a professionally driven administration, with an array of consulting bodies to support accountability that reach beyond the employee and employer confederations now controlling IMSS and that fail to represent the beneficiary base. Integration would also require health system regulation through truly national, universal institutions performing effectively across public and private actors.

It is still too early to tell the direction that the health system will take under President Andrés Manuel López Obrador for the years ahead. The focus of his campaign was on strengthening the public health system and discontinuing the financial architecture that characterizes the SPSS. However, it is possible that a focus on the public nature of the health system can be interpreted in terms of strengthening public financing and regulation, while enabling integration across public institutions and with the private sector. This is the key question to address in the early period of the new administration.

Response to the COVID-19 pandemic

As of 4 June 2020, Mexico reported 101 238 confirmed COVID-19 infection cases and 11 729 deaths from COVID-19, placing the country among the top 14 globally for numbers of cases and number 7 for deaths (Worldometer, 2020). The first case was confirmed on 24 March and, at the time of writing, the daily numbers of cases were still on an upward trend. Social distancing measures were introduced 24 March 2020; these were originally set to last until 30 April but were officially extended nationwide until the end of May when restrictions would be gradually lifted, based on federal and state guidelines, on the way towards a "new normality". Social distancing measures include the mandatory closure of non-essential businesses and in some states transportation restrictions to curtail movement. However, Mexico City has prolonged stricter social distancing measures in place at least until mid-June 2020 (NAO, 2020).

■ The economic impacts of the pandemic will be major

Economic growth has been projected to decline between 4.6% and 8.8% for 2020 due to COVID-19, while 686 000 formal sector jobs – those affiliated to IMSS – were lost in March and April 2020 (Banco de México, 2020), representing 3.3% of total employees at the end of 2019 (IMSS, 2019). However, the active labour force had been reduced by 12.3% by March, mostly due to social distancing measures affecting the informal sector (INEGI, 2020). Up to 12.2 million people have been projected to fall into poverty during 2020, with half of these falling into extreme poverty (Székely, Acevedo & Flores, 2020).

The administration of President López Obrador has introduced a few measures to address the immediate economic impact of the COVID-19 pandemic. In addition to strengthening existing social programmes directed to the poor, the government offered microcredit for the self-employed registered with IMSS, meeting low demand (Carvajal, 2020). The administration declined to inject liquidity into the economy, stating that small to large businesses should look after themselves and that the government should not incur any debt. To reduce the pandemic's impact on poverty, however, some experts suggest the government should spend at least 0.7% of GDP on targeted measures such as salary subsidies, postponement of fiscal obligations, unemployment insurance, strengthening social programmes and increasing microcredit (Székely Acevedo & Flores, 2020).

■ Monitoring and surveillance of the pandemic has been fraught with controversy

Mexico is using the sentinel model recommended by the Pan American Health Organization (PAHO) for the monitoring of respiratory diseases, but there are data limitations accompanied by a poor communication strategy. Established in 2006 and used for the H1N1 (swine flu) pandemic in 2009, this model is based on a sample of 475 hospitals and primary care units, including major public providers as well as some private providers (PAHO, 2014). Reporting is slow and provides information to the federal government with estimates that are reported at state level only and that are insensitive to local situations (NAO, 2020). In spite of daily news conferences by the vice minister for Prevention and Health Promotion of the MoH, the limitations of the data with respect to reporting delays and completeness were not properly communicated, which has led to confusion among the public regarding the actual numbers of cases and fatalities, as well as trends in the pandemic. Furthermore, failure to meet official expectations with regard to the date of the peak and the intensity of the pandemic, as well as premature statements regarding success in its control, added to uncertainty.

The number of tests carried out to confirm COVID-19 infection have been among the lowest in the world, with 1910 per million population, compared with 4104 in Brazil and upwards of 20 000 in countries with similar incomes such as Peru and Turkey (Worldometer, 2020). The federal government has focused testing on the most severe hospital cases, often confirming cases postmortem. This testing policy is likely to have contributed to Mexico being officially reported among countries of the world with highest lethality for COVID-19, at 10.7% of all cases, compared with 8.5% in Ecuador and 6.2% in Brazil – with far more cases than Mexico – and as low as 1% in Chile (Worldometer, 2020). In spite of recommendations by scientists and experts (Red ProCienciaMx, 2020), the government is maintaining its current surveillance policy, although efforts are being made to make more tests available.

■ ## Hospital capacity was reinforced through two main strategies: hospital strengthening and expansion of access

Public hospital capacity was bolstered by adding temporary beds, dedicating beds to COVID-19 and hiring additional personnel. While no figures have been published on new beds, just over 6500 physicians and 12 600 nurses were hired on a temporary basis, yet most of these were substituting for personnel with underlying health conditions and risks who were placed on temporary leave. Expansion of patient access to health care was undertaken mainly by freeing-up access to IMSS, Army and Navy hospitals regardless of affiliation.

To date, no decree or law has been established to facilitate and coordinate a system-wide response to address COVID-19. Social insurance and the MoH institutions, as well as hospitals, responded on a case-by-case basis, depending on bed availability. In some COVID-19-designated hospitals, beds and human resources were separated for the care of the insured and non-insured or were restricted to IMSS affiliates (Sánchez, 2020; IMSS, 2020), with greater integration in hospitals dedicated to non-COVID-19-related care. No specific financial arrangements have been announced; IMSS assured its workers through a specific agreement that their rights would be fully respected and promised a 20% salary bonus for front-line workers. Payment for non-beneficiary care would be sought from the federal government, although no specific financial mechanisms or fees were announced (IMSS, 2020). Anecdotal evidence suggests that non-affiliates were still being rejected in some hospitals (Martínez & Herrera, 2020), while no specific policies were announced; for example, in the case of ISSSTE or Pemex hospitals.

Private hospitals were at first threatened with a decree forcing them to provide free supplies of services as needed and with the potential imposition of government management. An agreement was eventually signed with two hospital chains to provide care for a list of non-COVID-19-related conditions payed for on the basis of a government-set schedule. These private hospitals made about 10% of their total private bed capacity available, amounting to 3.8% of that of the public sector. Notably, however, participating private hospitals are located in large urban centres and offer little service provision to the poor and to the population residing in smaller cities.

The supply of sexual and reproductive health services by public providers during the COVID-19 pandemic was addressed through a guideline to ensure continued provision, yet these services were not included in the agreement with the private sector. It can be expected that the impoverishing out-of-pocket expenditure will increase, contributing to the pandemic-related economic downturn (NAO, 2020).

Public hospital capacity came close to being overwhelmed by COVID-19 patients. There were also reports of patients forced to seek care at several COVID-19-designated hospitals prior to being accepted (Ricardo, 2020). Furthermore, one in five COVID-19 cases (Kitroeff & Villegas, 2020) and 3.1% of deaths affected health workers, a rate that is fivefold that in the United Kingdom (Cook & Kursumovic, 2020). This dire situation was accompanied by widespread health worker demonstrations demanding personal protection equipment.

Policy reflections

The response to COVID-19 brought to a crisis point the economic, social and health policy limitations that have affected Mexico for decades. The pandemic brought the health system to critical capacity exacerbating and exposing to a wide audience its many governance, infrastructure and technical limitations. As with all crises, the fight against infectious and chronic diseases and health risks has provided a tremendous opportunity to move decidedly forward in the future.

The health system was brought to its knees by the pandemic and will need time to recover. Health, social and economic policies will need to be formulated in a coordinated manner to ensure funding for health in the mid-term and to assure all citizens and investors that the pandemic is controlled and that the economy can be reinvigorated. Institutional segmentation should be eliminated in the short term to ensure equity through establishing a single door of entry to all regardless of contributions and to integrate health funding into a national purse capable of stimulating quality and efficiency.

The pandemic has highlighted the importance of all-of-government health policies making the most out of ever reduced resources. It is the time to reconceptualize the patchwork nature of universal health coverage in Mexico, to ensure that all citizens have effective access to quality health services and can better benefit from health risk protection through environmental and community protections and services.

9

Appendices

9.1 **References**

Abel-Smith B (1992). The Beveridge Report: its origins and outcomes. Int Soc Secur Rev.45:1–2.

Aldana A, Reyes A (2019). *Características sociodemográficas, acceso y condiciones de salud de los migrantes mexicanos en Estados Unidos y de retorno a México* [Sociodemographic characteristics, access and health status of Mexican migrants in the United States and on their return to Mexico]. In: Secretariat of the Interior/National Population Council (CONAPO). Migración y Salud/Migration and Health. México City: Secretariat of the Interior/National Population Council (CONAPO).

AMFEM (2016). *Directorio de Facultades y Escuelas Afiliadas* [Directory of Affiliated Faculties and Schools] [website]. Mexico City: AMFEM Asociación Mexicana de Facultades y Escuelas de Medicina, AC. (http://www.amfem.edu.mx/index.php/directorio, accessed 9 April 2020).

Amuedo Dorantes C, Sainz T, Pozo S (2007). Remittances and healthcare expenditure patterns of populations in origin communities: Evidence from Mexico. Washington, DC: Inter-American Development Bank.

ANFEM (2018). *COMAEM Consejo Mexicano para la Acreditación de la Educación Médica* [Mexican Council for the Accreditation of Medical Education]. Mexico City: AMFEM Asociación Mexicana de Facultades y Escuelas de Medicina, AC. (http://www.amfem.edu.mx/docs/2018/comaem.pdf, accessed 9 April 2020).

ANAFAM (2018). *Asociación Nacional de Fabricantes de Medicamentos, AC* [National Association of Drug Manufacturers, AC] [website]. Mexico City: ANAFAM Asociación Nacional de Fabricantes de Medicamentos, AC. (www.anafam.org.mx/inicio, accessed 9 April 2020).

ANUIES (2017). *Anuarios Estadísticos de Educación Superior* [Higher Education Statistical Yearbooks] [website]. Mexico City:ANUIES Asociación Nacional de Universidades e Instituciones de Educación Superior. (http://www.anuies.mx/informacion-y-servicios/informacion-estadistica-de-educacion-superior/anuario-estadistico-de-educacion-superior, accessed 9 April 2020).

Arvizu J, Morales A (2016). *Se pronuncia Narro por fortalecer intercambio en instituciones de salud* [Narro expresses the need for strengthening exchanges across health institutions]. *El Universal*, 11 October.

Asociación Nacional de Hospitales Privados (2018). *Directorio de Miembros* [Directory of Members] [website]. Mexico City: Asociación Nacional de Hospitales Privados. (http://www.anhp.org.mx/directorio.php, accessed 9 April 2020).

Asociación Pro Personas con Parálisis Cerebral (2018). *Asociación Pro Personas con Parálisis Cerebral* [Association of People with Cerebral Palsy] [website]. (http//:apac.mx/en/, accessed 9 April 2020).

Astorga I et al. (2016). *10 años de Asociaciones Público–Privadas (APP) en salud en América Latina ¿Qué hemos aprendido?* [10 years of Public–Private Partnerships (PPP) in health in Latin America. What have we learned?]. Washington: IADB.

Auditoría Superior de la Federación (2016). *Las Reformas Estructurales: Hacia una Seguridad Social Universal* [Structural reforms: Towards universal social security]. Mexico City: Cámara de Diputados.

Azpiri López JR (2016). Observations in relation to myocardial infarction: Are there three different Mexicos? Medicina Universitaria.18(72):181–184.

Banco de México (2020). *Informe trimestral enero–marzo 2020.* [Quarterly Report Jaunary–March 2020]. Mexico City: Banco de México.

Banco Mundial (2015). *Tasa de mortalidad en un año (por cada 1 000 personas)* [One-year mortality rate (per 1 000 people)] [database]. Washington, DC: World Bank. (http://datos.bancomundial.org/indicador/SPDYNCDRTIN, accessed 3 October 2018).

Banco Mundial (2018a). *Tasa de mortalidad, adultos, mujeres (por cada 1 000 mujeres adultas)* [Mortality rate, adults, women (per 1 000 adult women)] [database]. Washington, DC: World Bank. (https://datos.bancomundial.org/indicador/SPDYNAMRTFE?locations=MX, accessed 3 October 2018).

Banco Mundial (2018b). *Tasa de mortalidad, adultos, varones (por cada 1 000 varones adultos)* [Mortality rate, adults, males (per 1 000 adult males)] [database]. Washington, DC: World Bank. (https://datos.bancomundial.org/indicador/SPDYNAMRTMA?end=2016&locations=MX&start=19861.4.2, accessed 3 October 2018).

Barraza Lloréns et al. (2015). *Carga económica de la diabetes mellitus en México* [Economic burden of diabetes mellitus in Mexico]. México DF: Funsalud, pp. 37–38.

Barrientos Gutiérrez T (2010). *Evaluación científico-técnica de la Ley General para el Control del Tabaco de México* [Scientific and technical evaluation of the General Law for Tobacco Control in Mexico]. *Salud Publica Mex.*52:S277–S282.

Bautista Arredondo S et al. (2014). *Análisis del uso de servicios ambulatorios curativos en el contexto de la reforma para la protección universal en salud en México* [Analysis of the use of outpatient curative services in the context of Universal Health Coverage reform in Mexico]. *Salud Pública Méx.*56(1):18.

Berenzon Gorn S et al. (2013). *Evaluación del sistema de salud mental en México: ¿Hacia dónde encaminar la atención?* [Evaluation of the mental health system in Mexico City: In which direction should care be directed?] *Rev Panam Salud Pública.*33(4):252–258.

Busse R, Schreyögg J, Gericke C (2007). Analyzing changes in health financing arrangements in high-income countries: A comprehensive framework approach. HNP Discussion Paper. Washington, DC: World Bank.

Cámara de Diputados del H. Congreso de la Unión (2012). *Reglamento de la Ley General para el Control del Tabaco (2009)*. [Regulation of the General Tobacco Control Law (2009)]. *Última reforma publicada DOF-09-10-2012.* Mexico City: Gobierno de México. (http://www.conadic.salud.gob.mx/pdfs/reglamento_control_tabaco.pdf, accessed 11 June 2020).

Cámara de Senadores de los Estados Unidos Mexicanos (2008). *Ley General para el Control del Tabaco* [General Tobacco Control Law]. *Gaceta Oficial del Senado de la República.*198: 115–123.

Campos Navarro R, Peña Sánchez EY, Paulo Maya A (2017). *Aproximación crítica a las políticas públicas en salud indígena, medicina tradicional e interculturalidad en México (1990–2016)* [Critical approximation to public policies on indigenous health, traditional medicine and intercultural relations in Mexico (1990–2016)]. *Salud colectiva.*13(3):443–455.

Carvajal B (2020). *Microcréditos del IMSS van al fracaso.* [IMSS microcredits doomed to failure]. La Jornada, 14 May. (https://www.jornada.com.mx/ultimas/economia/2020/05/14/microcreditos-del-imss-van-al-fracaso-5356.html, accessed 8 June 2020).

Casar MA (2013). *Quince años de gobiernos sin mayoría en el Congreso mexicano* [Mexico: Fifteen years of minority governments (1997–2012)]. *Política y Gobierno*.XX(2):219–263. (http://www.scielo.org.mx/pdf/pyg/v20n2/v20n2a1.pdf, accessed 8 June 2020).

CCNPMIS Comisión Coordinadora para la Negociación de Precios de Medicamentos e Insumos para la Salud (2016). *Informe público al Ejecutivo Federal de los resultados de la Comisión* [Public report to the Federal Executive of the Commission's results]. Mexico City: s.n.

Centro Nacional para la Prevención de Accidentes Subsecretaría de Prevención y Promoción de la Salud (2011b). *Análisis de los Sistemas de Urgencias en México.* [Analysis of Emergency Care systems in Mexico]. Mexico City: Secretaría de Salud. (http://conapra.salud.gob.mx/Interior/Documentos/Publicaciones_Especializadas/Analisis_Sistemas_Urgencias.pdf, accessed 9 April 2020).

Centro Nacional para la Prevención y Control del VIH y el sida (2018). *Epidemiología/Registro Nacional de Casos de VIH y sida* [Epidemiology/National Registry of Cases of HIV and AIDS] [website]. Mexico City: Gobierno de México. (https://www.gob.mx/censida/documentos/epidemiologia-registro-nacional-de-casos-de-sida?idiom=es, accessed 9 April 2020).

CIA (2016). The World factbook. [website]. In: CIA/Library. Washington, DC: Central Intelligence Agency. (https://www.cia.gov/library/publications/the-world-factbook/rankorder/2147rank.html, accessed 8 June 2020).

Ciclo escolar (2018). *Los Estados y Capitales de México* [The States and Capitals of Mexico] [website]. Ciclo escolar. (https://www.cicloescolar.com/2012/06/los-estados-y-capitales-de-mexico.html, accessed 9 April 2020).

CIFRHS Comisión Interinstitucional para la Formación de Recursos Humanos para la Salud (2017). *XLI Examen Nacional para Aspirantes a Residencias Médicas 2017* [XLI National Examination for Aspirants to Medical Residences 2017] [website]. Mexico City: CIFRHS. (http://www.cifrhs.salud.gob.mx/site1/enarm/docs/2017/E41_plazas_mex_lugares_ext_2017.pdf, accessed 9 April 2020).

Cook T, Kursumovic E, (2020). Exclusive: Deaths of NHS staff from COVID-19 analysed. Health Service Journal, 22 April. (https://www.hsj.co.uk/simon-lennane/3008300.bio, accessed on 11 June 2020).

CNPSS Comisión Nacional de Protección Social en Salud (2013). *Informe de resultados del SPSS* [SPSS Results Report]. Mexico City: Secretaría de Salud.

CNPSS Comisión Nacional de Protección Social en Salud (2015). *Informe de resultados. Enero–junio de 2015* [Results report. January–June 2015]. Mexico City: Sistema de Protección Social en Salud.

CNPSS Comisión Nacional de la Protección Social en Salud (2018a). *Catálogo Universal de Servicios de Salud, CAUSES 2018* [Universal Health Services Catalog, CAUSES 2018]. Mexico City: Sistema de Protección Social en Salud.

CNPSS Comisión Nacional de Protección Social en Salud (2018b). *Informe de resultados. Enero–diciembre de 2018* [Results report. January–December 2018]. Mexico City: Sistema de Protección Social en Salud.

COFEPRIS (2016a). *Base de datos de licencias de fábricas de medicamentos alopáticos, homeopáticos, herbolarios* [License database for allopathic, homeopathic and herbal medicine factories] [website]. Mexico City: Gobierno de México. (https://www.gob.mx/cofepris/documentos/bases-de-datos-de-licencias-sanitarias-de-insumos-para-la-salud, accessed 9 June 2020).

COFEPRIS (2016b). *Verificación de farmacias con manejo de medicamentos controlados* [Verification of pharmacies with controlled medication management] [website]. Mexico City: Gobierno de México. (https://www.gob.mx/cofepris/acciones-y-programas/sistema-de-recetarios-electronicos-para-medicamentos-de-fraccion-i, accessed 9 June 2020).

COFEPRIS (2017). *COFEPRIS y la UNODC firman acuerdo para impulsar cuidados paliativos* [COFEPRIS and UNODC sign agreement to promote palliative care] [website]. Mexico City: Gobierno de México. (https://www.gob.mx/cofepris/prensa/cofepris-y-la-unodc-firman-acuerdo-para-impulsar-cuidados-paliativos, accessed 9 April 2020).

COFEPRIS (2018). *Guías, Lineamientos y Requerimientos de Farmacovigilancia* [Pharmacovigilance Guides, Guidelines and Requirements.] [website]. Mexico City: Gobierno de México. (https://www.gob.mx/cofepris/documentos/guias-lineamientos-y-requerimientos-de-farmacovigilancia, accessed 9 April 2020).

Colchero MA et al. (2015). Changes in prices after an excise tax to sweetened sugar beverages was implemented in Mexico City: Evidence from urban areas. PLOS One.10(12):e0144408. doi: 10.1371/journal.pone.0144408.

Colchero MA et al. (2017). Sustained consumer response: evidence from two-years after implementing the sugar sweetened beverage tax in Mexico. Health Aff (Millwood). 36(3):564–571. doi:10.1377/hlthaff.2016.1231.

Collins-Dogrul J (2006). Managing US–Mexico "border health": An organizational field approach. Soc Sci Med.63(12):3199–3211.

Comisión de Salud Fronteriza México–Estados Unidos (2017). *Comisión de Salud Fronteriza México–Estados Unidos, Sección México* [United States–Mexico Border Health Commission, Mexico Section] [website]. Mexico City: Comisión de Salud Fronteriza México–Estados Unidos. (http://www.saludfronterizamx.org/2017/es/acerca-comision/creacion, accessed 9 April 2020).

Comisión Federal de Competencia Económica (2017). *Estudio en materia de libre concurrencia y competencia sobre los mercados de medicamentos con patentes vencidas en México* [Study on the subject of free access and competition on markets of off-patent medicines]. Mexico City: COFECE.

CONACYT (2019). *La salud mental de los migrantes repatriados* [Mental health of repatriated migrants]. Mexico City: Consejo Nacional de Ciencia y Tecnología. (https://centrosconacyt.mx/objeto/la-salud-mental-de-los-migrantes-repatriados/ accessed 9 April 2020).

CONAMED (2008). *Factores de riesgo para la mala práctica. Análisis y aprendizaje por medio de resultados* [Malpractice risk factors. Results-based analysis and learning]. Mexico City: CONAMED.

CONAPO (2005). *Tasa de mortalidad infantil municipal* [Municipal infant mortality rate]. Mexico City: Consejo Nacional de Población.

CONAPO (2018a). *Indicadores demográficos de México de 1950 a 2050 y de las entidades federativas de 1970 a 2050* [Demographic indicators of Mexico from 1950 to 2050 and of the states from 1970 to 2050] [website]. Mexico City: Consejo Nacional de Población. (https://datos.gob.mx/herramientas/indicadores-demograficos-de-mexico-de-1950-a-2050-y-de-las-entidades-federativas-de-1970-a-2050?category=web&tag=economy, accessed 9 April 2020).

CONAPO (2018b). *Indicadores diversos 1990–2015* [Diverse indicators 1990–2015] [website]. Mexico City: Consejo Nacional de Población. (http://www.conapo.gob.mx/en/CONAPO/Indicadores, accessed 11 June 2020).

CONAPO (2018c). *Diccionario de las bases de datos de Proyecciones de la Población de México y las Entidades Federativas, 2016–2050* [Dictionary of Population Projection databases of Mexico and the Federal States, 2016–2050] [website]. Mexico City: Gobierno de México. (https://www.gob.mx/conapo/documentos/diccionario-de-las-bases-de-datos-de-proyecciones-de-la-poblacion-de-mexico-y-de-las-entidades-federativas-2016-2050, accessed 9 April 2020).

CONEVAL (2016). *Indicadores de carencia social, Estados Unidos Mexicanos, 2010–2015* [Indicators of social deprivation, United Mexican States, 2010–2015] [website]. Mexico City: CONEVAL. (https://www.coneval.org.mx/Medicion/EDP/Paginas/Datos-del-Modulo-de-Condiciones-Socioeconomicas.aspx, accessed 9 April 2020).

CONEVAL (2018). *Evaluación estratégica de protección social en México. Segunda Edición* [Strategic evaluation of social protection in Mexico, 2nd edn]. Mexico City: CONEVAL.

Connor SR, Sepulveda Bermedo MC, editors (2015). Global atlas on palliative care at the end of life. London: Worldwide Palliative Care Alliance.

Consejo de Ética y Transparencia de la Industria Farmacéutica (2009). *Códigos de la industria farmacéutica establecida en México* [Pharmaceutical codes of industries established in Mexico]. Mexico City: Cámara Nacional de la Industria Farmacéutica.

Consejo de Salubridad General (2015). *Certificación SiNaCEAM* [SiNaCEAM certification] [website]. Mexico City: Consejo de Salubridad General. (http://www.csg.gob.mx/contenidos/certificacion/sinaceam.html, accessed 9 April 2020).

Consejo Nacional Contra las Adicciones (2017). *Encuesta Nacional de Consumo de Drogas, Alcohol y Tabaco, ENCODAT 2016–2017* [National Survey of Drug, Alcohol and Tobacco Use, ENCODAT 2016–2017] [website]. Cuernavaca, Mexico City: INSP (https://www.gob.mx/salud%7Cconadic/acciones-y-programas/encuesta-nacional-de-consumo-de-drogas-alcohol-y-tabaco-encodat-2016-2017-136758, accessed 9 April 2020).

Consejo Nacional Contra las Adicciones et al. (2009). *Encuesta Nacional de Adicciones 2008* [2008 National Addiction Survey]. Cuernavaca, Mexico City: INSP.

Contreras Loya D, Reding Beltran A, Gómez Dantés O (2013). Evaluation of a comprehensive model for the treatment of hypertension, diabetes, and obesity in Mexico City: a retrospective longitudinal study. Lancet.381(S33). doi: 10.1016/S0140-6736(13)61287-8.

Córdova A (1972). *La formación del poder político en México* [The formation of political power in Mexico]. Mexico City: Ediciones Era.

Countryeconomy.com (2018). Canada: Life expectancy at birth [website]. Madrid: Alldatanow. (https://countryeconomy.com/demography/life-expectancy/canada?year=1964, accessed 11 June 2020).

de Guzman GC et al. (2007). A survey of the use of foreign-purchased medications in a border community emergency department patient population. J Emerg Med.33(2):213–221.

De la Fuente JR, Heinze Martin G (2014). *La enseñanza de la Psiquiatría en México* [Psychiatry Teaching in Mexico]. *Salud Mental*.37:523–530.

DGCES Dirección General de Calidad y Educación en Salud, Secretaría de Salud (2015). *Información de las Instituciones de Seguros Especializadas en Salud (ISES)* [Specialized Health Insurance Institutions Information (ISES)] [website]. Mexico City: Secretaría de Salud. (http://www.calidad.salud.gob.mx/site/regulacion/seguros_salud_instituciones.html, accessed 29 September 2018).

DGCES Dirección General de Calidad y Educación en Salud, Secretaría de Salud (2018). *Acreditación de Establecimientos y Servicios de Atención Médica* [Accreditation of Healthcare Facilities and Services] [website]. Mexico City: Secretaría de Salud. (http://www.calidad.salud.gob.mx/site/calidad/acreditacion.html, accessed 23 September 2018).

DGE Dirección General de Epidemiología, Secretaría de Salud (2016a). *Manual de Procedimientos Estandarizados para la Vigilancia Epidemiológica Hospitalaria* [Manual for Standardized Procedures for Hospital Epidemiological Surveillance]. Primera edición. Mexico City: Secretaría de Salud.

DGE Dirección General de Epidemiología, Secretaría de Salud (2016b). *Red Hospitalaria de Vigilancia Epidemiológica, Informe Anual 2015* [Hospital Network for Epidemiological Surveillance, Annual Report 2015]. Primera edición. Mexico City: Secretaría de Salud.

DGE Dirección General de Epidemiología, Secretaría de Salud (2018). *Anuario de Morbilidad 1984–2017. Incidencia por grupo de edad* [Morbidity yearbook 1984–2017. Incidence by age group] [database]. Mexico City: Secretaría de Salud. (http://www.epidemiologia.salud.gob.mx/anuario/html/incidencia_casos.html, accessed 9 April 2020).

DGIS (2015a). *Boletín de Información Estadística 2014–2015* [Statistical Information Bulletin 2014–2015]. Mexico City: Dirección General de Información en Salud, Secretaría de Salud. (http://www.dgis.salud.gob.mx/descargas/pdf/Boletxn_InformacixnEstadxstica_14_15.pdf, accessed on 26 September 2018).

DGIS (2015b). *Sistema de Cuentas en Salud a Nivel Federal y Estatal (SICUENTAS)* [Federal and State Health Accounts System (SICUENTAS)]. Mexico City: Dirección General de Información en Salud, Secretaría de Salud.

DGIS (2018a). *Recursos físicos y materiales (Infraestructura) 2003–2013* [Physical and material resources (Infrastructure) 2003–2013]. Mexico City: Dirección General de Información en Salud, Secretaría de Salud.

DGIS (2018b). *Catálogo Clave Única de Establecimientos de Salud (CLUES). Actualización Julio*

2018 [Catalog of health establishments' unique codes (CLUES). Update July 2018]. Mexico City: Dirección General de Información en Salud, Secretaría de Salud. (http://www.dgis. salud.gob.mx/contenidos/intercambio/clues_gobmx.html, accessed on 26 September 2018).

Diario Oficial de la Federación (1988). *Norma Técnica 321 para la Prevención del Retraso Mental producido por Hipotiroidismo Congénito* [Technical standard 321 for the prevention of mental retardation produced by congenital hypothyroidism]. Mexico City: Diario Oficial de la Federación, Órgano del Gobierno Constitucional de los Estados Unidos Mexicanos, Tomo CDXX, pp. 89–90.

Diario Oficial de la Federación (1995). *Ley del Seguro Social* [Social Security Law]. Mexico City: Diario Oficial de la Federación, Órgano del Gobierno Constitucional de los Estados Unidos Mexicanos, Tomo DVII, pp. 25–65.

Diario Oficial de la Federación (2003). *Decreto por el que se expide la Ley de Instituciones de Seguros y de Fianzas y se reforman y adicionan diversas disposiciones de la Ley sobre el Contrato de Seguro* [Decree by which the Law of Insurance Institutions and Bonds is issued and various provisions of the Law on the Insurance Contract are amended and added]. Mexico City: Diario Oficial de la Federación, Órgano del Gobierno Constitucional de los Estados Unidos Mexicanos, Tomo DCCXV, pp. 1–194.

Diario Oficial de la Federación (2007). *Decreto por el que se expide la Ley del Instituto de Seguridad y Servicios Sociales de los Trabajadores del Estado* [Decree by which the Law of the Institute of Security and Social Services of State Workers is issued]. Mexico City: Diario Oficial de la Federación, Órgano del Gobierno Constitucional de los Estados Unidos Mexicanos, Tomo DCXLII, pp. 2–64.

Diario Oficial de la Federación (2009). *Decreto por el que se reforma y adiciona la Ley General de Salud en Materia de Cuidados Paliativos* [Decree by which the General Health Law on Palliative Care is reformed and added]. Mexico City: Diario Oficial de la Federación. (http:// dof.gob.mx/nota_detalle.php?codigo=5076793&fecha=05/01/2009, accessed 9 April 2020).

Diario Oficial de la Federación (2013). *Norma Oficial Mexicana NOM-017-SSA2-2012, Para la vigilancia epidemiológica* [Official Mexican Standard NOM-017-SSA2-2012, For epidemiological surveillance]. Mexico City: Diario Oficial de la Federación. (http://dof. gob.mx/nota_detalle.php?codigo=5288225&fecha=19/02/2013, accessed 9 April 2020).

Diario Oficial de la Federación (2014). *Norma Oficial Mexicana NOM-011-SSA3-2014, Criterios para la atención de enfermos en situación terminal a través de cuidados paliativos* [Official Mexican Standard NOM-011-SSA3-2014, Criteria for terminally ill patient care through palliative care]. Mexico City: Diario Oficial de la Federación. (https://www.dof.gob.mx/nota_detalle. php?codigo=5375019&fecha=09/12/2014, accessed 9 April 2020).

Diario Oficial de la Federación (2016). *Acuerdo por el que se declara la obligatoriedad de los esquemas de manejo integral de cuidados paliativos, así como los procesos señalados en la Guía del Manejo Integral de Cuidados Paliativos en el Paciente Pediátrico* [Agreement declaring the obligation of comprehensive palliative care management schemes, as well as the processes outlined in the Guide to Comprehensive Palliative Care Management in Pediatric Patients]. Mexico City: Diario Oficial de la Federación. (http://www.dof.gob.mx/nota_detalle. php?codigo=5465444&fecha=14/12/2016, accessed 9 April 2020).

Diario Oficial de la Federación (2017a). *NORMA Oficial Mexicana NOM-220-SSA1-2016, Instalación y operación de la farmacovigilancia* [Official Mexican STANDARD NOM-220-SSA1-2016, Installation and operation of pharmacovigilance]. Mexico City: Diario Oficial de la Federación. (http://dof.gob.mx/nota_detalle.php?codigo=5490830&fecha=19/07/2017, accessed 9 April 2020).

Diario Oficial de la Federación (2017b). *EDICIÓN 2017 del Cuadro Básico de Medicamentos. Segunda y Tercera Sección* [2017 Edition of the Basic Table of Medicines. Second and Third Sections]. Mexico City: Diario Oficial de la Federación. (http://dof.gob.mx/nota_to_doc. php?codnota=5513536, accessed 9 April 2020).

Dirario Oficial de la Federación (2017c). *Reglamento interior de la comisión para definir tratamientos y medicamentos asociados a enfermedades que ocasionan gastos catastróficos* [Internal regulations of the commission to define treatments and medications associated with diseases causing catastrophic expenses]. Mexico City: Diario Oficial de la Federación. (https://dof.gob.mx/nota_detalle.php?codigo=5477656&fecha=27/03/2017, accessed 8 June 2020).

Díaz Ortega JL et al. (2012). *Cobertura de vacunación y proporción de esquema incompleto en niños menores de siete años en México* [Vaccination coverage and proportion of incomplete schedule in children under seven years of age in Mexico]. *Salud Publica Mex*.60(3):338–346.

Díaz Portillo SP et al. (2017). *Condiciones de trabajo en consultorios adyacentes a farmacias privadas en Mexico City: perspectiva del personal médico* [Working conditions in offices adjacent to private pharmacies in Mexico City: medical staff perspective]. *Gac Sanit*.31(6):459–465.

Doubova S et al. (2018). Loss of job-related right to healthcare is associated with reduced quality and clinical outcomes of diabetic patients in México. Int J Qual Health Care.30(4):283–290.

Dresser A et al. (2008). *Uso de antibióticos en México: revisión de problemas y políticas* [Antibiotic use in Mexico City: review of problems and policies]. *Salud Publica Mex*.50:S480–487.

Economou C (2010). Greece: Health system review. Health Syst Transit.12(7):1–180.

Economou C, Kaitelidou D, Karanikolos M, Maresso A. (2017) Greece: Health system review. Health Systems in Transition; 19(5):1–192. (http://www.euro.who.int/__data/assets/pdf_file/0006/373695/hit-greece-eng.pdf).

Fajardo Dolci G (2010). *La Comisión Nacional de Arbitraje Médico, sus antecedentes, su situación actual y futuro* [The National Medical Arbitration Commission, its background and its current and future situation]. Mexico City: CONAMED.

Fajardo Dolci G (2014). *Propuesta de modelo para la formación de médicos especialistas en México* [Proposal for a model for the training of medical specialists in Mexico]. In: G Fajardo Dolci, editor. *La formación de médicos especialistas en México* [The training of medical specialists in Mexico]. Mexico City: Academia Nacional de Medicina.

FAO (2017). FAOSTAT/New Food balances [database]. Rome: Food and Agriculture Organization of the United Nations. (http://www.fao.org/faostat/en/#data/FBS, accessed 3 October 2018).

Ferré F et al. (2014). Italy: Health System Review. Health Syst Trans.16(4):1–168.

Figueroa Lara A, González Block MA (2016). *Costo efectividad de una alternativa para la prestación de servicios de atención primaria en salud para los beneficiarios del Seguro Popular de México* [Cost effectiveness of an alternative for the provision of primary health care services for the beneficiaries of Mexico's Seguro Popular]. *Salud Pública Méx*.58:569–576.

Figueroa Lara A, González Block MA, Alarcón Irigoyen J (2016). Medical expenditure for chronic diseases in Mexico City: The case of selected diagnoses treated by the largest care providers. PloS One.11(1):e0145177.

Flores Echavarría R et al. (2001). *La formación médica en México y los procesos en búsqueda de garantizar la calidad de los egresados* [Medical training in Mexico and the processes in search of guaranteeing the quality of graduates]. *Rev Fac Med* UNAM.44(2):75–80.

Fraga Sastrías JM et al. (2010). *Sistemas médicos de emergencia en México. Una perspectiva prehospitalaria* [Emergency medical systems in Mexico. A prehospital perspective]. *Arch Med Urgen Méx*.2(1):25–34.

Frenk J (2010). The World Health Report 2000: Expanding the horizon of health system performance. Health Policy Plan.25:343–345. doi:10.1093/heapol/czq034.

Freyermuth G, Luna M, Muños JA (2014). *Indicadores 2014. Mortalidad materna en México* [Indicators 2014. Maternal mortality in Mexico]. Mexico City: CIESAS (http://www.omm.org.mx/images/stories/Documentos%20grandes/INDICADORES_2014_Web.pdf, accessed 9 April 2020).

Fundación Teletón (2015). *Rehabilitación e inclusión* [Teletón Childrens' rehabilitation and inclusion centre] [website]. (http://www.teleton.org/home/contenido/centro-de-rehabilitacion-infantil-teleton, accessed 9 June 2020).

Funsalud (2012). *Descripción del sector farmacéutico en México* [Description of the pharmaceutical sector in Mexico]. Mexico City: Fundación Mexicana para Salud.

Funsalud (2014). *Estudio sobre la práctica de la atención médica en consultorios médicos adyacentes a farmacias privadas* [Study on the practice of medical care in medical offices adjacent to private pharmacies]. Mexico City: Fundación Mexicana para Salud.

García Alonso EM (2015). *Evolución del nacimiento por cesárea: El caso de México* [Evolution of caesarean birth: The case of Mexico]. DILEMATA.18:27–43.

García Armesto S et al. (2010). Spain: Health system review. Health Syst Trans.12(4):1–295.

García Díaz R, Sosa-Rubí S (2011). Analysis of the distributional impact of out-of-pocket health payments: Evidence from a public health insurance program for the poor in Mexico. J Health Econ.30:707–718.

Gómez Dantés H et al. (2016). Dissonant health transition in the states of Mexico, 1990–2013: a systematic analysis for the Global Burden of Disease Study 2013. Lancet.388:2386–2402.

Gómez Dantés O et al. (2011). *Sistema de Salud de México* [Mexican health system]. *Salud Publica Mex.*53:S220–S232.

González Barrera A (2015). More Mexicans Leaving than coming to the US. In: Pew Research Center/ Hispanic trends [website]. Washington, DC: Pew Research Center. (http://www.pewhispanic.org/2015/11/19/more-mexicans-leaving-than-coming-to-the-u-s/, accessed 9 April 2020).

González Block MA (1990). *Génesis de los principios de organización en la salud pública de México* [Genesis of the principles of organization in public health in Mexico]. *Salud Pública Méx.*32:337–351.

González Block MA (2017). *¿Qué compra, cómo y de quién el Seguro Popular de México? Experiencia con la compra estratégica nacional y en una entidad pionera* [What, how and from whom does Mexico's Seguro Popular buy? Experience with national strategic purchases in a pioneering entity]. *Salud Pública Méx.*59:59–67.

González Block MA (2018). *El Seguro Social: evolución histórica, crisis y perspectivas de reforma* [Social Security: historical evolution, crisis and prospects for reform]. Mexico City: Universidad Anáhuac.

González Block MA, de la Sierra de la Vega LA (2011). Hospital utilization by Mexican migrants returning to mexico due to health needs. BMC Public Health.11:241.

González Block MA, López Santibáñez C (2011). *Evaluación de las estrategias de portabilidad y convergencia hacia la integración del Sistema Nacional de Salud* [Evaluation of the strategies of portability and convergence towards the integration of the National Health System]. Cuernavaca, México: INSP. (http://bit.ly/MSjG2m, accessed 9 June 2020).

González Block MA, Martínez González G (2015). *Hacia la cobertura universal de la protección financiera de la salud en México. Tendencias y oportunidades para la colaboración público–privada* [Towards universal coverage of financial health protection in Mexico. Trends and opportunities for public–private collaboration]. Mexico City: AMIS-Funsalud.

González Block MA et al. (2011). *Evaluación y estrategias de portabilidad y convergencia hacia la integración del sistema nacional de salud* [Evaluation and strategies of portability and convergence towards the integration of the national health system]. Mexico City: INSP.

González Block MA et al. (2012). Redressing the limitations of the Affordable Care Act for Mexican undocumented immigrants through bi-national health insurance: a willingness to pay study in Los Angeles. J Immigr Minor Health.16(2):179–188.

González Block MA et al. (2016). *Asignación financiera en el Sistema de Protección Social en Salud México: retos para la compra estratégica* [Financial allocation in Mexico's Social Protection System in Health: challenges for strategic purchasing]. *Salud Pública Méx.*58, 522–532.

González Block MA et al. (2018a). Decentralization of health policy and services in Mexico. In: Marchildon P, Bossert TJ. Federalism and decentralization in health care. A decision space approach. Toronto: Forum of Federations.

González Block MA et al. (2018b). *El subsistema privado de atención a la salud en México: Diagnóstico y retos, 1ª Edn.* [The private health care subsystem in Mexico: Diagnosis and challenges, 1st edn]. Mexico City: Universidad Anáhuac.

González Block MA et al. (2018c). *La separación de las funciones financieras y de prestación de servicios de salud en el Seguro Popular. Formulación, alcances y retos de la reforma del 4 de junio de 2014* [The separation of the financial functions and the provision of health services in Seguro Popular. Formulation, scope and challenges of the 4 June 2014 reform]. Mexico City: Comisión Nacional de Protección Social en Salud.

González Pier E (2008). *Política farmacéutica saludable* [Healthy pharmaceutical policy]. *Salud Publica Mex*.50:S488–495.

González Pier E, Barraza LM (2011). *Trabajando por la salud de la población: Propuestas de política para el sector farmacéutico* [Working for the health of the population: Policy proposals for the pharmaceutical sector]. Mexico City: Mexico City: Fundación Mexicana para Salud.

González Pier E et al. (2005). *Sistema de Protección Social en Salud. Elementos conceptuales, financieros y Operativos* [Social Protection System in Health. Conceptual, financial and operational elements]. Mexico City: Secretaría de Salud.

Grupo de trabajo de la Fundación Mexicana para la Salud (2013). *Universalidad de los servicios de salud en México* [Universality of health services in Mexico]. *Salud Pública Méx*.55: EE1–EE64.

Guerra G et al. (2018). Loss of job-related right to healthcare due to employment turnover: challenges for the Mexican health system. BMC Health Serv Res.8:457.

Gutiérrez G, González Block MA, Reyes H (2015). *Desafíos en la implantación de guías de práctica clínica en instituciones públicas de México. Estudio de casos múltiple* [Challenges in the implementation of clinical practice guidelines in public institutions in Mexico. Multiple case study]. *Salud Pública Méx*.57(6):547–554.

Gutiérrez J et al. (2011). *Los medicamentos genéricos: ¿Más barato por lo mismo?* [Generic drugs: the same thing cheaper?] *Elementos*.81:41–47.

Gutiérrez JP et al. (2012). *Encuesta Nacional de Salud y Nutrición 2012. Resultados Nacionales* [National Health and Nutrition Survey 2012. National Results]. Mexico City: INSP.

Gutiérrez P et al. (2016). *Monitoreo de la desigualdad en protección financiera y atención a la salud en México: análisis de las encuestas de salud 2000, 2006 y 2012* [Monitoring inequality in financial protection and health care in Mexico City: analysis of the 2000, 2006 and 2012 health surveys]. *Salud Pública Méx*.58(6):639–647.

Guzmán González JM (2016). *Presente y futuro de la rehabilitación en México* [Present and future of rehabilitation in Mexico]. *Cirugía y Cirujanos*.84(2):93–95.

Health Research Institute (2017). Top ten health industry issues of México: A whole-society approach to healthcare. Mexico City: PwC.

Heinze G, Chapa GC, Carmona-Huerta J (2016). *Los especialistas en psiquiatría en México: año 2016* [The specialists in psychiatry in Mexico City: year 2016]. *Salud Mental*.39(2):69–76.

Hernández López MF, Hernández Vázquez MR, Sánchez Castillo M (2013). *La salud sexual y reproductiva de las mujeres hablantes de lengua indígena, 1997–2009* [The sexual and reproductive health of Indigenous language-speaking women, 1997–2009]. In: CONAPO. *La situación demográfica de México 2013* [The demographic situation in Mexico 2013]. Mexico City: CONAPO.

Hospital Infantil de México Federico Gómez (2012). *Hospital Infantil de México Federico Gómez* [Federico Gómez Children's Hospital of Mexico]. Mexico City: Secretaría de Salud.

Ibarra I et al. (2013). *Capacidad del marco jurídico de las instituciones públicas de salud de México para apoyar la integración funcional* [Capacity of the legal framework of public health institutions in Mexico to support functional integration]. *Salud Pública Méx*.55(3):310–317.

IESM-OMS (2011). *Informe sobre el sistema de salud mental en México* [Report on the mental health system in Mexico]. Mexico City: Pan American Health Organization.

IHME (2018). Healthcare access and quality profiles. Seattle: Institute for Health Metrics and Evaluation. (http://www.healthdata.org/sites/default/files/files/county_profiles/HAQ/2018/Mexico_HAQ_GBD2016.pdf, accessed 9 April 2020).

IMSS (2020). *Pactan IMSS y Sindicato atención a pacientes COVID-19 no derechohabientes y respeto a derechos laborales.* [IMSS and Trade Unions agree on COVID-19 care for non-rights holder patients and respect to labour rights]. Mexico City: Instituto Mexicano del Seguro Social. (http://www.imss.gob.mx/prensa/archivo/202005/257, accessed 28 May 2020).

IMSS (2005). *El IMSS en Cifras. Las intervenciones quirúrgicas* [The IMSS in numbers. Surgical interventions]. *Rev Med Inst Mex Seguro Soc.*43(6):511–520.

IMSS (2014). *Informe al Ejecutivo Federal y al Congreso de la Unión sobre la Situación Financiera* [Report to the Federal Executive and the Congress of the Union on the Financial Situation]. Mexico City: Instituto Mexicano del Seguro Social.

IMSS (2017). *Informe al Ejecutivo Federal y al Congreso de la Unión sobre la Situación Financiera* [Report to the Federal Executive and the Congress of the Union on the Financial Situation]. Mexico City: Instituto Mexicano del Seguro Social.

IMSS (2018). *Nota Informativa. La compra consolidada de medicamentos 2017–2018* [Informative note. The consolidated purchase of medicines 2017–2018]. Mexico City: Instituto Mexicano del Seguro Social.

IMSS (2019). *En 2019 se crearon 342 mil empleos* [In 2019 343 thousand employment positions were created]. Mexico City: Instituto Mexicano del Seguro Social. (http://www.imss.gob.mx/prensa/archivo/202001/020, accessed on 28 May 2020).

IMSS (2020). *IMSS recibe primeros pacientes COVID-19 en hospital de expansión Autódromo Hermanos Rodríguez* [IMSS receives the first COVID-19 patients in the expansion hospital Autódromo Hermanos Rodríquez]. Mexico City: Instituto Mexicano del Seguro Social. (http://www.imss.gob.mx/prensa/archivo/202005/290, accessed 5 June, 2020).

INAPAM (2016). *Albergues y Residencias de día Inapam* [Inapam hostels and residences] [website]. Mexico City: Gobierno de México. (https://www.gob.mx/inapam/acciones-y-programas/albergues-y-residencias-diurnas-inapam, accessed 9 April 2020).

INAPAM (2014). *INAPAM promueve en sus albergues, Modelos de Atención Gerontológica* [INAPAM promotes Gerontological Care Models in its shelters] [website]. Mexico City: Gobierno de México. (https://www.gob.mx/inapam/prensa/inapam-promueve-en-sus-albergues-modelos-de-atencion-gerontologica, accessed 9 April 2020).

INDRE (2015). *Criterios de operación para la Red Nacional de Laboratorios de Salud Pública. Componente Vigilancia Epidemiológica. Versión No. 01* [Operation criteria for the National Network of Public Health Laboratories. Epidemiological Surveillance Component. Version No. 01]. Mexico City: Instituto Nacional de Referencia Epidemiológica.

INEGI (nd). *Extensión territorial* [Territorial extent of Mexico] In: INEGI/Cuantame [website]. Mexico City: Instituto Nacional de Estadística y Geografía. (http://cuentame.inegi.org.mx/territorio/extension/default.aspx?tema=T, accessed 8 June 2020).

INEGI (nd). *Indicadores por entidad federativa* [Indicators by state]. In: INEGI/Datos [website]. Mexico City: Instituto Nacional de Estadística y Geografía. (https://www.inegi.org.mx/app/estatal/, accessed 8 June 2020).

INEGI (2018). Encuesta Nacional de Salud y Nutrición 2018. Presentación de resultados. [National Health and Nutrition Survey 2018. Presentation of results]. Mexico City, INEGI. (https://www.inegi.org.mx/contenidos/programas/ensanut/2018/doc/ensanut_2018_presentacion_resultados.pdf, accessed 11 June 2020).

INEGI (2003). *La evolución de los hogares unipersonales* [The evolution of one-person households]. Mexico City: Instituto Nacional de Estadística y Geografía.

INEGI (2005). *Climatología* [Climatology]. Mexico City: Instituto Nacional de Estadística y Geografía. Mexico City: Instituto Nacional de Estadística y Geografía. (https://www.inegi.org.mx/temas/climatologia/, accessed 11 June 2020).

INEGI (2015). *Encuesta Intercensal 2015* [Intercensal Survey 2015]. In: INGEI/Programas [website]. Mexico City: Instituto Nacional de Estadística y Geografía. (https://www.inegi.org.mx/programas/intercensal/2015/, accessed 8 June 2020).

INEGI (2016a). *Encuesta Nacional de Ingresos y Gastos de los Hogares, 2016* [National Survey of Household Income and Expenses, 2016]. Mexico City: Instituto Nacional de Estadística y Geografía. (https://www.inegi.org.mx/programas/enigh/nc/2016/, accessed 11 June 2020).

INEGI (2016b). *Recursos para la salud. Estadísticas por tema* [Resources for health. Statistics by topic]. Mexico City: Instituto Nacional de Estadística y Geografía. (http://www3.inegi. org.mx/sistemas/sisept/default.aspx?t=msal37&s=est&c=22512, accessed 2 October 2018).

INEGI (2016c). *Trabajo no remunerado de los hogares* [Unpaid households' work] [website]. Mexico City: Instituto Nacional de Estadística y Geografía. (https://www.inegi.org.mx/ temas/tnrh/, accessed 11 June 2020).

INEGI (2017b). *Estadísticas a propósito de la industria farmacéutica, 2017* [Statistics on the pharmaceutical industry, 2017]. Mexico City: Instituto Nacional de Estadística y Geografía. (https://codigof.mx/estadisticas-a-proposito-la-industria-farmaceutica/, accessed 9 April 2020).

INEGI (2017c). *Estadísticas a propósito del Día de las y los cuidadores de personas dependientes (2 de marzo). Datos Nacionales* [Statistics relevant for the Day of the Caregivers of Dependent People (March 2). National Data] [website]. Mexico City: Instituto Nacional de Estadística y Geografía. (http://www.diputados.gob.mx/sedia/biblio/usieg/comunicados/25ene19/ economia/9_cuidadoresdepersonasdependientes_230118-9.pdf, accessed 11 June 2020).

INEGI (2017d). Road traffic accidents in urban and suburban areas [website]. Mexico City: Instituto Nacional de Estadística y Geografía. (https://www.inegi.org.mx/programas/ accidentes/, accessed 11 June 2020).

INEGI (2018a). *Banco de Indicadores* [Indicators Bank] [website]. Mexico City: Instituto Nacional de Estadística y Geografía. (https://www.inegi.org.mx/app/indicadores/, accessed 11 June 2020).

INEGI (2018b). *Características educativas de la población* [Population educational characteristics] [website]. Mexico City: Instituto Nacional de Estadística y Geografía. (https://www.inegi. org.mx/temas/educacion/, accessed 11 June 2020).

INEGI (2019). *Estadísticas a propósito del día mundial para la prevención del suicidio (10 de septiembre). Datos nacionales* [Statistics on the World Prevention of Suicide day (September 10). National data]. Mexico City: Instituto Nacional de Estadística y Geografía. (https:// www.inegi.org.mx/contenidos/saladeprensa/aproposito/2019/suicidios2019_Nal.pdf, accessed 8 June 2020).

INEGI (2020). *Resultados de la encuesta telefónica de ocupación y empleo (ETOE) cifras oportunas de abril de 2020* [Results of the Telephone Occupation and Employment survey (ETOE). Early results for April 2020]. Mexico City: Instituto Nacional de Estadística y Geografía. (https://www.inegi.org.mx/contenidos/saladeprensa/boletines/2020/enoe_ie/ETOE.pdf, accessed 11 June 2020).

INSP (2012). *Encuesta Nacional de Salud y Nutrición 2012. Vacunación en niños: hacia un mejor registro y la aplicación sin restricciones* [National Health and Nutrition Survey 2012. Vaccination in children: towards better registration and unrestricted application]. Mexico City: Instituto Nacional de Salud Pública.

INSP (2013). *Regulación de la Publicidad de Alimentos y bebidas no alcohólicas en México: El Código PABI vs. Regulaciones Internacionales* [Regulation of Advertising of Food and non-alcoholic beverages in Mexico City: The PABI Code vs. International regulations] [website]. Mexico City: Instituto Nacional de Salud Pública. (https://www.insp.mx/epppo/blog/2865-reg-publicidad- alimentos-bebidas-mex-codigo-pabi-vs-reg-intern-439.html, accessed 9 April 2020).

INSP (2018a). *Informe encuestoteca* [Report of the survey library] [website]. Mexico City: Instituto Nacional de Salud Pública. (https://www.insp.mx/centros/evaluacion-y-encuestas/ uisp/encuestoteca.html, accessed 11 June 2020).

INSP/CIESAS (2008). External evaluation of opportunities,1997–2007; 10 years of $$. Mexico City: Instituto Nacional de Salud Pública, Centro de Investigación y Estudios en Superiores en Antropología Social.

Instituto Mexicano de la Propiedad Industrial (2017). *Mes de la lucha contra el cáncer de mama* [Fight against breast cancer month] [website]. Mexico City: Gobierno de México. (https:// www.gob.mx/impi/articulos/mes-de-la-lucha-contra-el-cancer-de-mama, accessed 9 April 2020).

Instituto Nacional de las Mujeres (2012). *El trabajo de cuidados: ¿Responsabilidad compartida?* [Care work: shared responsibility?]. Mexico City: Gobierno de México. (https://evaluacionyseguimientoproyectosindesol.wordpress.com/2015/07/13/inmujeres-sf-el-trabajo-de-cuidados-responsabilidad-compartida/, accessed 11 June 2020).

ISSSTE Instituto de Seguridad y Servicios Sociales de los Trabajadores del Estado (2014). *Curso de apoyo para cuidadores informales de personas envejecidas frágiles y con demencia* [Support course for informal caregivers of fragile and demented aged people] [website]. Mexico City: Gobierno de México. (http://www.issste.gob.mx/cursocuidadores2/, accessed 9 April 2020).

Jiménez-Ornelas RA, Cardiel-Téllez L (2013). *El suicidio y su tendencia social en México: 1990–2011* [Suicide and its social tendency in Mexico City: 1990–2011]. *Papeles Poblac.*19(77): 205–223.

Kitroeff N, Villegas P (2020). "It's not the virus": Mexico's broken hospitals become killers, too. New York Times, 28 May.

Knaul F, Frenk J (2005). Health insurance in México: Achieving universal coverage through structural reform. Health Aff.24(6):1467–1476.

Knaul FM, Arreola Ornelas H, Méndez Carniado O (2016). *Protección financiera en salud: actualizaciones para México a 2014* [Financial protection in health: updates for Mexico to 2014]. *Salud Pública Méx.*58:341–350.

Knaul FM et al. (2012). The quest for universal health coverage: achieving social protection for all in México. Lancet.380(9849).1259–1279.

Landeck M, Garza C (2002). Utilization of physician health care services in Mexico by US Hispanic border residents. Health Mark Q.20(1):3-16.

Lozano R et al. (2013). *Evaluación externa del Fondo de Protección Contra Gastos Catastróficos del Sistema de Protección Social de la Salud 2013* [External evaluation of the Fund for Protection Against Catastrophic Expenditures of the Social Health Protection System 2013]. Mexico City: Instituto Nacional de Salud Pública.

Macías JL (2005). *Geología e historia eruptiva de algunos de los grandes volcanes activos de México* [Geology and eruptive history of some of the great active volcanoes in Mexico]. *Bol Soc Geol Mex.*57(3):45.

Martínez C, Herrera R (2020). *Sufren contagiados saturación en CDMX.* [Infected suffer saturation in Mexico City]. Reforma, 12 May.

Martínez Martínez M et al. (2012). Health research funding in Mexico City: The need for a long-term agenda. Plos One.7(12):e51195.

Martínez Valle A, Molano Ruíz M, editors (2013). *El México del 2013. Propuesta para transformar el Sistema Nacional de Salud* [México in 2013. Proposal to transform the National Health System]. Mexico City: Centro de Estudios Espinosa Yglesias.

Médicos Sin Fronteras (2019). *Jóvenes afectados por la violencia, sin atención en salud mental en México* [Youth affected by violence, without mental health care in Mexico]. Mexico City: Médicos Sin Fronteras. (https://www.msf.mx/article/jovenes-afectados-por-la-violencia-sin-atencion-en-salud-mental-en-mexico, accessed 9 April 2020).

Medina Mora M et al. (2007). Psychiatric disorders in Mexico City: lifetime prevalence in a nationally representative sample. Br J Psychiatry.190:521–528.

Medina Mora ME (2003). *Prevalencia de trastornos mentales y uso de servicios: Resultados de la Encuesta Nacional de Epidemiología Psiquiátrica en México* [Prevalence of mental disorders and use of services: Results of the National Survey of Psychiatric Epidemiology in Mexico]. *Salud Mental.*26:1–16.

Mir Cervantes C (2016). *Evaluación Formativa para el programa "El Médico en tu Casa" de la Secretaría de Salud del Distrito Federal: evaluaciones de diseño, procesos e interacción con el usuario. Informe Final* [Formative Evaluation for the "The Doctor in your House" programme of the Federal District Health Secretariat: evaluations of design, processes and interaction with users. Final report]. Mexico City: Centro de Investigación y Docencia Económicas AC (CIDE).

Moreno EM, López JC, García CC (2016). *Las compras consolidadas de medicamentos: ¿Una política pública de salud eficiente?* [Consolidated drug purchases: An efficient public health policy?] *Revista Legislativa de Estudios Sociales y de Opinión Pública.*9(18):47–103.

Movimiento de Regeneración Nacional (2018). *Proyecto de Nación 2018–2024* [2018–2024 Project for the Nation]. Mexico City: MORENA.

Muñoz Hernández O (2006). *Programas Integrados de Salud (PREVENIMSS)* [Integrated Health Programmes (PREVENIMSS)]. *Rev Med Inst Mex Seguro Soc.*44:S1–S2.

Murayama Rendón C, Ruesga Benito SM (2016). *Hacia un Sistema Nacional Público de Salud en México* [Towards a National Public Health System in Mexico]. Mexico City: UNAM Programa Universitario de Estudios del Desarrollo.

Narro Robles J, Cordera Campos R, Lomelí Venegas L (2006). *Hacia la Universalización de la Seguridad Social* [Towards the Universalization of Social Security]. Mexico City: UNAM.

Narro Robles J, Moctezuma Navarro D, Orozco Hernández L (2010). *Hacia un nuevo modelo de seguridad social* [Towards a new model of social security]. *EconomíaUNAM.*7(número especial):7–33.

Nava I (2016). *La economía de los hogares unipersonales en México* [The economy of one-person households in Mexico]. In: CONAPO. *La situación demográfica de México 2015* [The demographic situation of Mexico 2015]. Mexico City: Consejo Nacional de Población. (http://www.conapo.gob.mx/es/CONAPO/La_economia_de_los_hogares_unipersonales_en_Mexico, accessed 9 April 2020).

North American Health Systems Observatory (NAO) (2020). North American COVID-19 policy response monitor. Toronto: University of Toronto. (https://ihpme.utoronto.ca/research/research-centres-initiatives/nao/covid19/, accessed 11 June 2020).

Observatorio de Mortalidad Materna en México (2018). Numeralia 2016. Mortalidad materna en México. Mexico City, Centro de Investigaciones y Estudios Superiores en Antropología Social. (https://omm.org.mx/wp-content/uploads/2020/04/Numeralia-2016.pdf, accessed 11 June 2020).

OECD (2016). *Estudios de la OCDE sobre los Sistemas de Salud: México 2016* [OECD Studies on Health Systems: Mexico 2016]. Paris: OECD.

OECD (2017a). How's Life? 2017. Measuring well-being. Paris: OECD.

OECD (2017b). Health at a Glance 2017: OECD Indicators. Paris: OECD.

OECD (2018a). Gross fixed capital formation in the health care system [database]. Paris: OECD. (https://stats.oecd.org/Index.aspx?DataSetCode=SHA_HK, accessed 29 September 2018).

OECD (2018b). Health care expenditure and financing. Paris: OECD. (https://stats.oecd.org/Index.aspx?DataSetCode=SHA#, accessed 20 September 2018).

OECD (2018c). Health statistics [database]. Paris: OECD. (https://stats.oecd.org/index.aspx?queryid=30183#, accessed on 27 September 2018).

OECD (2018d). Life expectancy at birth [database]. Paris: OECD. (https://data.oecd.org/healthstat/life-expectancy-at-birth.htm, accessed 2 November 2018).

OECD (2018e). Family database. Age of mothers at childbirth and age-specific fertility [database]. Social Policy Division – Directorate of Employment, Labour and Social Affairs. Paris: OECD. (http://www.oecd.org/els/family/database.htm, accessed 8 June 2020).

OECD (2018f). Income inequality. In: OECD data [website]. Paris: OECD (https://data.oecd.org/inequality/income-inequality.htm, accessed 8 June 2020).

OECD (2019). Health status [database]. Paris: OECD. (https://stats.oecd.org/index.aspx?DataSetCode=HEALTH_STAT#, accessed on 27 September 2018).

Oficina de Información Científica y Tecnológica para el Congreso de la Unión (2018). *Nota Número 007* [Note number 007]. Mexico City: Congreso de México.

OPS (2013). *Informe sobre los sistemas de salud mental en América Latina y el Caribe* [Report on mental health systems in Latin America and the Caribbean]. Washington, DC: Organización Panamericana de la Salud.

OPS (2017). *Encuesta Global de Tabaquismo en Adultos. México 2015* [Global Survey of Smoking in Adults. Mexico 2015]. Cuernavaca, México: Instituto Nacional de Salud Pública / Organización Panamericana de la Salud.

Ordorica Mellado M (2014). *1974: Momento crucial de la política de población* [1974: Crucial moment of population policy]. *Papeles Poblac.*20(81).9–23.

Oxman A et al. (2010). A framework for mandatory impact evaluation to ensure well informed public policy decisions. Lancet.375:427–431.

PAHO (2014). Operational guidelines for sentinel severe acute respiratory infection (SARI) surveillance. Washington,DC: Pan American Health Organization.

Pastrana T et al. (2012). *Atlas de Cuidados Paliativos en Latinoamérica ALCP* [Palliative Care Atlas in Latin America ALCP]. Houston: IAHPCPress.

Peña Nieto E (2017). *Quinto Informe de Gobierno* [Fifth Government Report]. Mexico City: Presidencia de la República.

Perdigón Villaseñor G, Fernández Cantón SB (2008). *Principales causas de muerte en la población general e infantil en México, 1922–2005* [Main causes of death in the general and child population in Mexico, 1922–2005]. *Bol Med Hosp Infant Mex.*65(3):238–240.

Perez Cuevas R et al. (2015). A social health services model to promote active ageing in Mexico City: design and evaluation of a pilot programme. Ageing Soc.35(7):1457–1480.

Presidencia de la República (2018). *Garantizar abasto de medicamentos suficientes, de calidad y a precios accesibles ha sido prioridad en la política social del presidente EPN* [Ensuring the supply of sufficient, quality and affordable medicines has been a priority in President EPN's social policy] [website]. Mexico City: Gobierno de México. (https://www.gob. mx/presidencia/prensa/garantizar-abasto-de-medicamentos-suficientes-de-calidad-y-a-precios-accesibles-ha-sido-prioridad-en-la-politica-social-del-presidente-epn, accessed 11 June 2020).

PrevenISSSTE (2020). *PrevenISSSTE Cerca de ti* [PrevenISSSTE close to you] [website]. Mexico City: Gobierno de México. (https://prevenissstecercadeti.wordpress.com/prevenissste/, accessed 9 April 2020).

Procuraduría Federal del Consumidor (2006). *Precios máximos en medicamentos* [Maximum prices on medicines]. Mexico City: Procuraduría Federal del Consumidor. (https://www.profeco. gob.mx/encuesta/brujula/bruj_2006/pdf06/2006-01-09%20Precios%20m%C3%A1mos%20 %20dicamentos.pdf, accessed 11 June 2020).

Ramiro HM et al. (2017). *El ENARM y las escuelas y facultades de medicina. Un análisis que no le va a gustar a nadie* [The ENARM and the schools and faculties of medicine. An analysis that no one will like]. *Rev Med Inst Mex Seguro Soc.*55(4):498–511.

Red ProCienciaMx (2020). *Científicos piden acciones de contención urgentes para proteger a la población de México durante la pandemia y ofrecen colaboración.* [Scientists request urgent contention actions to protect the population of Mexico during the pandemic and offer their collaboration]. (https://twitter.com/ProCienciaMx/status/1241116745403957248, March 20; www.bit.ly/396wi3V, accessed 11 June 2020).

Reynales Shigematsu LM et al. (2017). *Instituto Nacional de Psiquiatría Ramón de la Fuente Muñiz; Instituto Nacional de Salud Pública, Comisión Nacional Contra las Adicciones, Secretaría de Salud. Encuesta Nacional de Consumo de Drogas, Alcohol y Tabaco 2016–2017: Reporte de Tabaco* [National Survey of Consumption of Drugs, Alcohol and Tobacco 2016–2017: Tobacco Report]. Mexico City: INPRFM.

Ricardo J (2020). *Muere por Covid-19 tras recorrer 7 hospitales* [Dies from COVID-19 after visiting 7 hospitals]. Reforma, 14 May.

Roberts MJ, Hsiao WC, Reich MR (2015). Disaggregating the Universal Coverage cube: putting equity in the picture. Health Syst Ref.1(1):22–27.

Rodríguez CE (2016). *El Sistema Nacional de Investigadores en números* [The National System of Researchers in numbers]. Mexico City: Foro Consultivo Científico y Tecnológico, AC.

Rubio Monteverde H, Rubio Monteverde TM, Álvarez Cordero R (2011). *Impacto de las políticas antitabaco en México* [Impact of anti-smoking policies in Mexico]. *Rev Fac Med UNAM.*54(5):22–33.

Salgado N et al. (in press). Migrant health vulnerability through the migration process: Implications for health policy in Mexico and the United States. In: Latapí E, Lowell L, Martin S, *Diálogo Binacional sobre Migrantes Mexicanos en Estados Unidos y México*. Washington DC: CIESAS, Georgetown University.

Saludiario (2016). *Ley obliga a especialistas a obtener certificación médica: CONAMED* [The law obliges specialists to obtain medical certification: CONAMED]. *Saludiario*, 25 October.

Sánchez ME (2020). *Admite director del IMSS errores en Monclova* [IMSS hospital admits mistakes in Monclova]. Reforma, 25 April.

Santa Ana Tellez Y et al. (2013). Impact of over-the-counter restrictions on antibiotic consumption in Brazil and Mexico. Plos One.8(10):e75550.

Santacruz Varela J et al. (2015). *Metodología para estimar el número de médicos especialistas en México* [Methodology to estimate the number of medical specialists in Mexico]. In: Fajardo Dolci G editor. *La Formación de Médicos Especialistas en México* [The Training of Specialist Doctors in Mexico]. Mexico City: Academia Nacional de Medicina, pp. 89–94.

Saturno Hernández PJ et al. (2017). *Implementación de indicadores de calidad de la atención en hospitales públicos de tercer nivel en México* [Implementation of quality of care indicators in third level public hospitals in Mexico]. *Salud Publica Mex*.9:227–235.

Saturno PJ et al. (2014). *Calidad del primer nivel de atención de los servicios estatales de salud. Diagnóstico estratégico de la situación actual* [Quality of the first level of care of state health services. Strategic diagnosis of the current situation]. Cuernavaca: INSP-BID, pp. 20.

Secretaría de Comercio (2017). *Precios registrados de medicamentos con patente vigente* [Registered prices of medicines with current patent] [website]. Mexico City: Gobierno de México. (http://www.economia.gob.mx/files/transparencia/focalizada/precios_medicina_de_patente_noviembre_2017.pdf, accessed 11 June 2020).

Secretaría de Economía. Unidad de Inteligencia de Negocios (2016). *Diagnóstico sectorial* [Sectoral diagnosis]. Mexico City: PROMÉXICO.

Secretaría de Gobernación (2012). *Manual de Organización General de la Secretaría* [General Ministerial Organization Handbook] [website]. Mexico City: Secretaría de Gobernación. (https://dof.gob.mx/nota_detalle.php?codigo=5264646&fecha=17/08/2012, accessed 9 April 2020).

Secretaría de Relaciones Exteriores (2016). *Instituto de los Mexicanos en el Exterior* [Institute of Mexicans Abroad] [website]. Mexico City: Secretaría de Relaciones Exteriores. (https://www.gob.mx/sre/acciones-y-programas/instituto-de-los-mexicanos-en-el-exterior, accessed 11 June 2020).

Secretaría de Salud (1995). *Norma Oficial Mexicana NOM-007-SSA2-1993. Atención de la mujer durante el embarazo, parto y puerperio y recién nacido. Criterios y procedimientos para la prestación del servicio* [Mexican Official Standard NOM-007-SSA2-1993. Care of women during pregnancy, childbirth and puerperium and the newborn. Criteria and procedures for the provision of the service]. Mexico City: Diario Oficial de la Federación Órgano del Gobierno Constitucional de los Estados Unidos Mexicanos Tomo CDXCVI; pp. 19–38.

Secretaría de Salud (1999). *Norma Oficial Mexicana NOM-167-SSA-1997, para la prestación de servicios de asistencia social para menores y adultos mayores* [Official Mexican Standard NOM-167-SSA-1997, for the provision of social assistance services for minors and older adults]. Mexico City: Diario Oficial de la Federación Órgano del Gobierno Constitucional de los Estados Unidos Mexicanos. (http://www.salud.gob.mx/unidades/cdi/nom/167ssa17.html, accessed 27 August 2018).

Secretaría de Salud (2001). *Programa de Acción en Salud Mental* [Mental Health Action Programme]. Mexico City: Secretaría de Salud.

Secretaría de Salud (2005). *Hacia una política farmacéutica integral para México* [Towards a comprehensive pharmaceutical policy for Mexico]. Mexico City: Secretaría de Salud.

Secretaría de Salud (2007a). *Programa de acción específico 2007–2012. Vete Sano, Regresa Sano* [Specific action programme 2007–2012. Go healthy, come back healthy]. Mexico City: Secretaría de Salud.

Secretaría de Salud (2007b). *Programa de Acción Específico 2007–2012. Medicina Tradicional y Sistemas Complementarios de Atención a la Salud* [Specific Action Programme 2007–2012. Traditional Medicine and Complementary Health Care Systems]. Mexico City: Secretaría de Salud.

Secretaría de Salud (2009a). *Reglamento de la Ley General para el Control del Tabaco* [Regulation of the General Law for Tobacco Control]; 31 de Mayo de 2009; Diario Oficial de la Federación.

Secretaría de Salud (2009b). *NOM-045-SSA2-2005 Vigilancia, prevención y control de las infecciones nosocomiales* [NOM-045-SSA2-2005 Surveillance, prevention and control of nosocomial infections]. Mexico City, Mexico City: Diario Oficial de la Federación Órgano del Gobierno Constitucional de los Estados Unidos Mexicanos.

Secretaría de Salud (2011). *Manual de lineamientos para el intercambio de servicios en el sector salud* [Handbook of Guidelines for the exchange of services in the health sector]. Mexico City: Secretaría de Salud.

Secretaría de Salud (2012a). *Convenio general de colaboración para la atención de la emergencia obstétrica* [General collaboration agreement for obstetric emergency care]. Mexico City: Secretaría de Salud.

Secretaría de Salud (2012b). *Norma Oficial Mexicana NOM-017-SSA3-(2012). Regulación de servicios de salud para la práctica de la acupuntura humana y métodos relacionados.* [Mexican Official Standard NOM-017-SSA3- (2012). Health services regulation for the practice of human acupuncture and related methods]. Mexico City: Diario Oficial de la Federación Órgano del Gobierno Constitucional de los Estados Unidos Mexicanos, Secretaría de Salud.

Secretaría de Salud (2013a). *Observatorio de los Servicios de Atención Primaria (2012).* [Observatory of Primary Care Services (2012)]. Mexico City: Dirección General del Evaluación del Desempeño. Secretaría de Salud.

Secretaría de Salud (2013b). *Programa de Acción Específico: Vacunación Universal 2013–2018* [Specific Action Program: Universal Vaccination 2013–2018] [website]. Mexico City: Secretaría de Salud. (http://www.censia.salud.gob.mx/contenidos/descargas/transparencia/especiales/PAE_Vacunacion_Universal_PAE_final_final.pdf, accessed 9 April 2020).

Secretaría de Salud (2013c). *Programa de Acción Específico Salud Mental (PAE) 2013–2018* [Specific Action Programme Mental Health (PAE) 2013–2018]. Mexico City: Secretaría de Salud.

Secretaría de Salud (2013d). *Programa de Acción Específico Prevención, Detección y Control de los Problemas de Salud Bucal 2013–2018* [Specific Action Programme Prevention, Detection and Control of Oral Health Problems 2013–2018]. Mexico City: Secretaría de Salud.

Secretaría de Salud (2013e). *Programa sectorial de salud 2013-2018* [Health sector programme 2013–2018]. Mexico City: Secretaría de Salud.

Secretaría de Salud (2014a). *Programa de Acción Específico: Sistema Nacional de Vigilancia Epidemiológica 2013–2018* [Specific Action Programme: National Epidemiological Surveillance System 2013–2018]. Mexico City: Secretaría de Salud. (https://www.gob.mx/cms/uploads/attachment/file/211946/PAE_2013-2018.pdf, accessed 9 April 2020).

Secretaría de Salud (2014b). *Norma Oficial Mexicana NOM-013-SSA2-2014 Para la prevención y control de enfermedades bucales* [Official Mexican Standard NOM-013-SSA2-2014 for the prevention and control of oral diseases]. Mexico City: Diario Oficial de la Federación Órgano del Gobierno Constitucional de los Estados Unidos Mexicanos, Secretaría de Salud.

Secretaría de Salud (2014c). *Puebla pone en marcha estrategias para acercar los servicios de salud a la población indígena* [Puebla implements strategies to bring health services closer to the indigenous population] [website]. Mexico City: Secretaría de Salud. (https://www.gob.mx/salud/prensa/puebla-pone-en-marcha-estrategias-para-acercar-los-servicios-de-salud-a-la-poblacion-indigena, accessed 9 April 2020).

Secretaría de Salud (2015a). *Dirección General de Epidemiología: Sistema Nacional de Vigilancia Epidemiológica* [General Directorate of Epidemiology: National Epidemiological Surveillance System] [website]. Mexico City: Secretaría de Salud. (https://www.gob.mx/

salud/acciones-y-programas/direccion-general-de-epidemiologia-sistema-nacional-de-vigilancia-epidemiologica, accessed 22 September 2018).

Secretaría de Salud (2015b). *Modelo de Atención Integral de Salud (MAI). Documento de Arranque* [Comprehensive Health Care Model (MAI)]. Startup Document]. Mexico City: Secretaría de Salud.

Secretaría de Salud (2015c). *Avanza el uso de Telesalud o Telemedicina en México* [The use of telehealth or telemedicine is advancing in Mexico] [website]. Mexico City: Secretaría de Salud. (https://www.gob.mx/salud/prensa/avanza-el-uso-de-la-telesalud-o-telemedicina-en-mexico, accessed 9 April 2020).

Secretaría de Salud (2015d). *Sistema de Cuentas en Salud a Nivel Federal y Estatal (Sicuentas)* [System of Health Accounts at Federal and State Level (Sicuentas)]. Mexico City: Secretaría de Salud.

Secretaría de Salud (2016a). *Acciones y Programas* [Actions and Programmes] [website]. Mexico City: Secretaría de Salud. (https://www.gob.mx/salud/es/archivo/acciones_y_programas, accessed 11 June 2020).

Secretaría de Salud (2016b). *Informe sobre la Salud de los Mexicanos 2016. Diagnóstico general del Sistema Nacional de Salud* [Report on the Health of Mexicans 2016. General diagnosis of the National Health System]. Mexico City: Secretaría de Salud.

Secretaría de Salud (2018a). *Secretaría de Salud* [Health Ministry] [website]. Mexico City: Secretaría de Salud. (https://www.gob.mx/salud/#395, accessed 11 June 2020).

Secretaría de Salud (2018b). *Conmemoración Día Internacional del Cáncer Infantil* [International Childhood Cancer Day Commemoration] [website]. Mexico City: Secretaría de Salud. (https://www.gob.mx/salud/acciones-y-programas/conmemoracion-dia-internacional-del-cancer-infantil, accessed 11 June 2020).

Secretaría de Salud (2019). *Programa sectorial de salud 2019–2024* [Health sector programme 2019–2024]. Mexico City: Secretaría de Salud.

Secretaría particular del Jefe de Gobierno (2017). *Quinto informe de gobierno de la Ciudad de México* [Fifth Mexico City government report]. Mexico City: CDMX.

Senado de la República (2016). *Avala Comisión de Salud declarar el 9 de agosto como Día Nacional de Lucha Contra el Cáncer Cervicouterino* [The Health Commission endorses August 9 as the National Day of the Fight Against Cervical Cancer] [website]. Mexico City: Senado de la República. (http://comunicacion.senado.gob.mx/index.php/informacion/grupos-parlamentarios/32754-avala-comision-de-salud-declarar-el-9-de-agosto-como-dia-nacional-de-lucha-contra-el-cancer-cervicouterino.html, accessed 9 April 2020).

Shama Levy T et al. (2016). *Encuesta Nacional de Salud y Nutrición de Medio Camino 2016. Informe Final de Resultados* [Midway National Health and Nutrition Survey 2016. Final Results Report]. Mexico City: Secretaría de Salud–Instituto Nacional de Salud Pública.

Sistema Nacional DIF (2016). *Centros de Rehabilitación* [Rehabilitation centres] [website]. Mexico City: Gobierno de México. (https://www.gob.mx/difnacional/acciones-y-programas/centros-de-rehabilitacion, accessed 11 June 2011).

STPS (2018). *Estadísticas sobre Accidentes y Enfermedades de Trabajo 2017* [Statistics on work accidents and diseases 2017] [website]. (http://autogestionsst.stps.gob.mx/Proyecto/Content/pdf/Estadisticas/Nacional.pdf, accessed 11 June 2020).

Székely M, Acevedo I, Flores I (2020). *Magnitud del impacto social del COVID-19 en México, y alternativas para amortiguarlo* [Magnitude of the social impact of COVID-19 in Mexico, and alternatives to cushion it]. Mexico City: Centro de Estudios Educativos y Sociales CEES.

Temores Alcántara G et al. (2015). *Salud mental de migrantes centroamericanos indocumentados en tránsito por la frontera sur de México* [Mental health of undocumented Central American migrants in transit along the southern border of Mexico]. *Salud Publica Mex*.57:227–233.

Transparency International (2018). *Corruption Perception Index 2017* [database]. Berlin: Transparency International. (https://www.transparency.org/news/feature/corruption_perceptions_index_2017#tableTransparency, accessed 11 June 2020).

Trigo Madrid M et al. (2014). *Resultados del Programa de Tamiz Neonatal Ampliado y epidemiología perinatal en los servicios de sanidad de la Secretaría de Marina Armada de México* [Results of the Expanded Neonatal Screening Programme and perinatal epidemiology in the health services of the Secretariat of the Navy of Mexico]. *Acta Pediat Mex*.35:448–458.

Uscanga Sánchez S et al. (2014). *Indicadores del proceso de tamizaje de cáncer de mama en México: un estudio de caso* [Indicators of breast cancer screening process in Mexico City: a case study]. *Salud Pública Méx*.56(5)528–537.

Vega RA (2019). *La migración médica como forma de acceder a la atención médica en el Valle del Río Grande* [Medical migration as a way to access medical care in the Rio Grande Valley]. In: Secretariat of the Interior/National Population Council (CONAPO). Migración y Salud / Migration and Health. México City: Secretariat of the Interior/National Population Council (CONAPO).

Velázquez E, Iturralde Nieto G (2012). *Afrodescendientes en México. Una historia de silencio y discriminación* [People of African descent in Mexico. A story of silence and discrimination]. Mexico City: Consejo Nacional para Prevenir la Discriminación.

Velázquez Ramírez MC (2017). *Se firma convenio de investigación entre el IMSS, COFEPRIS y la industria farmacéutica* [Research agreement signed between IMSS, COFEPRIS and the pharmaceutical industry]. *Código F*, 19 January.

Villatoro Velázquez A et al. (2017). *Encuesta Nacional de Consumo de Drogas, Alcohol y Tabaco 2016–2017: Reporte de Tabaco.* [National Survey of Consumption of Drugs, Alcohol and Tobacco 2016–2017: Tobacco report]. Mexico City: INPRFM.

Wallace S, Mendez Luck C, Castañeda X (2009). Heading south: Why Mexican immigrants in California seek health services in Mexico. Med Care.47(6):662–669.

Wirtz VJ, Dresser A, Heredia Pi I (2013). *Retos y oportunidades para el desarrollo de la política farmacéutica nacional en México* [Challenges and opportunities for the development of the national pharmaceutical policy in Mexico]. *Salud Publica Mex*.55(3):329–336.

WHO (2001). How to develop and implement a national drug policy: Updates and replaces Guidelines for Developing National Drug Policies, 1988, 2 edn. Geneva: World Health Organization.

Worldometer (2020). COVID-19 coronavirus pandemic [website]. (https://www.worldometers. info/coronavirus/?utm_campaign=homeAdvegas1?%22%20%5Cl%20, accessed on 28 May 2020).

World Bank (2018). World Bank Open Data. [database]. Washington, DC: World Bank. (https://data.worldbank.org/, accessed 3 October 2018).

Yarza de De la Torre E (2003). *Los volcanes del Sistema Volcánico Transversal* [The volcanoes of the transverse volcanic system]. Investigaciones Geográficas, Boletín del Instituto de Geografía, UNAM.50:220–234.

Zolla C (2007). *La salud de los pueblos indígenas de México* [The health of the indigenous peoples of Mexico]. Mexico City: DR National Autonomous University of Mexico. (http://www. nacionmulticultural.unam.mx/portal/pdf/proyectos_academicos/salud_pueblos_indigenas. pdf, accessed 8 June 2020).

Zong J, Batalova J (2016). Mexican immigrants in the United States [website]. Washington, DC: Migration Policy Institute. (https://www.migrationpolicy.org/article/mexican-immigrants-united-states, accessed 9 April 2020).

9.2 **Useful websites**

INSTITUTION NAME	INITIALS	URL
Federal Commission for the Protection Against Sanitary Risks	COFEPRIS	https://www.gob.mx/cofepris
Institute for Social Security and Services for State Employees	ISSSTE	https://www.gob.mx/issste
Mexican Association of Innovative Pharmaceutical Industry	AMIIF	https://amiif.org
Mexican Petroleum Company	PEMEX	https://www.pemex.com
Mexican Social Insurance Institute	IMSS	http://www.imss.gob.mx
Ministry of Health	SSA	https://www.gob.mx/salud
National Academy of Medicine	ANM	http://anmm.org.mx/
National Chamber of the Pharmaceutical Industry	Canifarma	http://www.canifarma.org.mx/
National Commission for Institutes of Health and High Specialty Hospitals	CINSHAE	https://www.gob.mx/insalud
National Council for the Evaluation of Social Development Policy	CONEVAL	https://www.coneval.org.mx/Paginas/principal.aspx
National Council on Population	CONAPO	https://www.gob.mx/conapo
National Institute of Statistics and Geography	INEGI	https://www.inegi.org.mx/
National Insurance and Securities Commission	CNSF	https://www.gob.mx/cnsf
National System for Integral Family Development	DIF	https://www.gob.mx/difnacional

9.3 **HiT methodology and production process**

HiTs are produced by country experts in collaboration with the Observatory's research directors and staff. They are based on a template that, revised periodically, provides detailed guidelines and specific questions, definitions, suggestions for data sources and examples needed to compile reviews. While the template offers a comprehensive set of questions, it is intended to be used in a flexible way to allow authors and editors to adapt it to their particular national context. The latest version of the template (2019) is available on the Observatory website http://www.euro.who.int/__data/assets/pdf_file/0009/393498/hit-template-eng.pdf?ua=1

Authors draw on multiple data sources for the compilation of HiTs, ranging from national statistics, national and regional policy documents to published literature. Furthermore, international data sources may be incorporated, such as those of the OECD and the World Bank. The OECD Health Data contain over 1200 indicators for the 34 OECD countries. Data are drawn from information collected by national statistical bureaux and health ministries. The World Bank provides World Development Indicators, which also rely on official sources.

In addition to the information and data provided by the country experts, the Observatory supplies quantitative data in the form of a set of standard comparative figures for each country, drawing on the European Health for All database. The Health for All database contains more than 600 indicators defined by the WHO Regional Office for Europe for the purpose of monitoring Health in All policies in Europe. It is updated for distribution twice a year from various sources, relying largely upon official figures provided by governments, as well as health statistics collected by the technical units of the WHO Regional Office for Europe. The standard Health for All data have been officially approved by national governments.

HiT authors are encouraged to discuss the data in the text in detail, including the standard figures prepared by the Observatory staff, especially if there are concerns about discrepancies between the data available from different sources.

A typical HiT consists of nine chapters.

1. Introduction: outlines the broader context of the health system, including geography and sociodemography, economic and political context, and population health.
2. Organization and governance: provides an overview of how the health system in the country is organized, governed, planned and regulated, as well as the historical background of the system; outlines the main actors and their decision-making powers; and describes the level of patient empowerment in the areas of information, choice, rights and cross-border health care.
3. Financing: provides information on the level of expenditure and the distribution of health spending across different service areas, sources of revenue, how resources are pooled and allocated, who is covered, what benefits are covered, the extent of user charges and other out-of-pocket payments, voluntary health insurance and how providers and health workers are paid.

4. Physical and human resources: deals with the planning and distribution of capital stock and investments, infrastructure and medical equipment; the context in which IT systems operate; and human resource input into the health system, including information on workforce trends, professional mobility, training and career paths.

5. Provision of services: concentrates on the organization and delivery of services and patient flows, addressing public health, primary care, secondary and tertiary care, day care, emergency care, pharmaceutical care, rehabilitation, long-term care, services for informal carers, palliative care, mental health care and dental care.

6. Principal health reforms: reviews reforms, policies and organizational changes; and provides an overview of future developments.

7. Assessment of the health system: provides an assessment of systems for monitoring health system performance, the impact of the health system on population health, access to health services, financial protection, health system efficiency, health care quality and safety, and transparency and accountability.

8. Conclusions: identifies key findings, highlights the lessons learned from health system changes; and summarizes remaining challenges and future prospects.

9. Appendices: includes references and useful websites.

The quality of HiTs is of real importance since they inform policy-making and meta-analysis. HiTs are the subject of wide consultation throughout the writing and editing process, which involves multiple iterations. They are then subject to the following.

- A rigorous review process.
- There are further efforts to ensure quality while the report is finalized that focus on copy-editing and proofreading.
- HiTs are disseminated (hard copies, electronic publication, translations and launches).

The editor supports the authors throughout the production process and in close consultation with the authors ensures that all stages of the process are taken forward as effectively as possible.

One of the authors is also a member of the Observatory staff team and they are responsible for supporting the other authors throughout the writing and production process. They consult closely with each other to ensure that all stages of the process are as effective as possible and that HiTs meet the series standard and can support both national decision-making and comparisons across countries.

■ 9.4 **The review process**

This consists of three stages. Initially the text of the HiT is checked, reviewed and approved by the series editors of the European Observatory. It is then sent for review to two independent academic experts, and their comments and amendments are incorporated into the text, and modifications are made accordingly. The text is then submitted to the relevant ministry of health, or appropriate authority and policy-makers within those bodies are restricted to checking for factual errors within the HiT.

■ 9.5 **About the authors**

Miguel Á González Block graduated in Natural Sciences and Social Anthropology from the University of Cambridge; doctorate from El Colegio de México in Social Sciences with a specialization in Sociology. Researcher and Professor of Anáhuac University and National Institute of Public Health, Mexico. Research interests include reforms of national health systems towards universal coverage and the capacity to use best evidence in health systems decision-making.

Lucero Cahuana Hurtado graduated with a Bachelor of Science degree in Economics, Peruvian Pontifical Catholic University; Master of Science degree in Health Economics, Center of Economics Teaching and Research, Mexico; Doctorate in Health Systems Research, National Institute of Public Health of Mexico. Professor at the School of Public Health and Administration at Cayetano Heredia University of Peru. Research interests include health financing, health systems, and health economics.

Hortensia Reyes Morales graduated as a Medical Doctor, National Autonomous University of Mexico; Doctorate in Sciences in Health Systems, National Institute of Public Health, Mexico. Interested in quality of health care; and health services evaluation and in care innovation design and evaluation.

Alejandra Balandrán Medical Doctor, Public Health Specialist, Master's in Public Health Administration, PhD Candidate in Health Policy. Technical Coordinator of Clinical Excellence, Instituto Mexicano del Seguro Social. Research interests include health systems, social inequalities in health, primary care, quality of health care, evidence-based public health, and integrated health service delivery networks.

Edna Madaí Méndez Hernández graduated as a Medical Doctor from Juárez University of Durango, Mexico, where she also obtained her Doctorate in Medical Sciences. Head of the Postgraduate Studies Department at the National Institute of Genomic Medicine (INMEGEN). Research interests include health care quality and nosocomial infection prevention.

INDEX

Note: Tables are indicated by a t appended to page numbers and figures are indicated by an f.

accessibility, 179–81, 186
accidents, traffic (motor vehicle), 11, 12t, 13, 15t, 47
accountability and transparency, 176–7
accreditation, 50t, 61, 63–4, 119, 122, 139, 171–2
acupuncture, 157
acute myocardial infarction (AMI), 14, 30, 184
acute otitis media, 15, 16t
addictions, 15, 47, 54, 57, 126, 128, 137
adolescents: overweight and obesity, 131, 186; physical activity, 13; responsibility for, 126; teen pregnancy and reproductive health, 46, 126, 184. *See also* children
African Mexicans, 2
ageing, demographic, 1, 4
Aguascalientes, 105t, 114f, 117f, 161
AIDS. *See* HIV/AIDS
alcohol consumption, 14, 15t
Alemán, Miguel, 25
allocative efficiency, 187–8
alternative and complementary medicine, 156–7
ambulance services, 141–2
ambulatory care, 43, 50–1t, 98, 124, 135–6
Ambulatory Care Medical Units, 136
AMEGI (Mexican Association of Interchangeable Generic Medicines), 68
AMFEM (Mexican Association of Faculties and Schools of Medicine), 119, 120
AMH (Mexican Association of Hospitals), 64
AMIIF (Mexican Association of Innovative Pharmaceutical Industry), 67, 68

ANADIM (National Association of Drug Distributors), 145t
anaemia, 14
ANAFAM (National Association of Pharmaceutical Manufacturers), 68, 144
ANAFARMEX (National Association of Pharmacies of Mexico), 145t
ANEFAR (National Association of Regional Pharmaceutical Companies), 145t
ANHP (National Association of Private Hospitals), 64
ANM (National Academy of Medicine), 19, 111, 122
APAC (Association for the Support of People with Cerebral Palsy), 149
Apprende (app), 110
apps, 108, 110
Archives of Biomedical Research (journal), 179
ASE (state government solidary contribution), 60
ASF (*Aportación Solidaria Federal;* federal solidary contribution), 60, 92
ASFed (General Audit of the Federation), 61
assessment, of health system, 175–89; summary, 175–6; accessibility, 179–81; acute medical care, 139–40; efficiency, 187–9, 187f; financial protection, 181–2; Healthcare Access and Quality (HAQ) Index, 182, 183f; health information systems, 179; infant mortality, 185; life expectancy, 185; outcomes, 185–7; performance monitoring and research, 178–9; public participation, 177; quality, 184–5; transparency and accountability, 176–7

Association for the Support of People with Cerebral Palsy (APAC), 149

asthma, 15, 16t

Atlantic Charter, 23

Automated Hospital Discharge Subsystem (SAEH), 48

Avila Camacho, Manuel, 23, 25

Baja California: general physicians, 114f; hospital beds, 105t; medical education, 120; medical specialists, 117f; municipalities, 6; specialty hospital co-ownership in, 39

Baja California Sur: general physicians, 114f; health spending inequalities, 161; hospital beds, 105t, 106; medical education, lack of, 119; medical specialists, 117f; municipalities, 6; population, 2

Beveridge Report, 23

birth rate, 3t

breast cancer, 12t, 126, 132, 137, 165, 180

bronchopneumonia, 15, 16t

caesarean births, 184

Calderón Hinojosa, Felipe, 30, 41, 166

Calles, Plutarco E, 21, 22

CAMOHM (Centre for Social Care of the Health of Older Adults), 141

Campeche: general physicians, 114, 114f; health system outcomes, 186; hospital beds, 105t, 106; medical specialists, 117f; population, 2

cancer: generic drugs and, 147; health promotion campaigns, 132; mammograms and mammograph equipment, 108t, 186; responsibility for cervical and breast cancer, 126; types of: breast, 12t, 126, 132, 137, 165, 180; cervical, 12t, 126, 132, 186; prostate, 12t

Canifarma (National Chamber of the Pharmaceutical Industry), 67–8

Cardenas, Lazaro, 22–3

cardiovascular diseases. *See* acute myocardial infarction; ischaemic heart disease

career paths, in health professions, 122–3

caregivers: informal, 151; for long-term care, 150–1

Carlos Slim Foundation (FCS), 47, 110, 130

cash transfers, conditional, 29, 46

catastrophic expenditures, 29, 35, 159, 160, 161t, 162, 163, 175, 181, 181f, 191. *See also* Protection Fund for Catastrophic Health Expenditures (FPGC)

CAUSES (Universal Health Services Catalogue), 35, 61, 62, 90, 139, 146, 154, 163

CCPNMIS (Coordinating Commission for Negotiating the Price of Medicines and other Health Inputs), 41, 66

CENETEC (National Centre of Technological Excellence in Health), 65

CENSIA (National Centre for the Health of Children and Adolescents), 126

CENSIDA (National Centre for the Prevention and Control of HIV/AIDS), 126

centralization, of health system, 43–5, 166, 170

Centre for Social Care of the Health of Older Adults (CAMOHM), 141

cerebrovascular diseases, 11

cervical cancer, 12t, 126, 132, 186

CETIFARMA (Council for Ethics and Transparency of the Pharmaceutical Industry), 67, 123

CFM (Mexican Pharmaceutical Consortium), 67, 68

Chiapas: complementary and alternative medicine, 157; general physicians, 114f; Healthcare Access and Quality (HAQ) Index, 182; health system outcomes, 186; hospital beds, 105t, 106; medical specialists, 116, 117f; social development, 10

chickenpox, 15, 16t

Chihuahua, 105t, 114f, 117f

children: cancer health promotion, 132; child delivery, 186; infant mortality, 2, 10t, 11, 185; neonatal screening, 128, 129–30; overweight and obesity, 13, 131; paediatric palliative care, 152; rehabilitation, 149; responsibility for, 126; sexual abuse, 46; vaccinations, 129, 132, 186. *See also* adolescents

cholera, 131

chronic obstructive pulmonary disease (COPD), 14

CIFRHS (Interinstitutional Commission for the Training of Human Resources for Health), 111–12

CINSHAE (National Commission for National Institutes of Health and High Specialty Hospitals), 34, 36, 111, 138
cirrhosis, alcohol, 11, 14
clinical practice guidelines (CPGs), 168
CLUES (Unique Health Establishment Code), 48
CMM (National College of Physicians, 64, 110–11
CNDH (National Commission for Human Rights), 68
CNPSS (Commission for Social Protection in Health), 35, 37, 44, 59, 60–1, 70, 90, 92, 98, 177
Coahuila de Zaragoza, 105t, 114f, 117f
COFECE (Federal Commission for Economic Competition), 66, 147
COFEPRIS. *See* Federal Commission for the Protection Against Sanitary Risks (COFEPRIS)
Colima, 2, 105t, 114f, 117f, 161, 187
COMAEM (Mexican Council for Accreditation of Medical Education), 119
Commission for Social Protection in Health (CNPSS), 35, 37, 44, 59, 60–1, 70, 90, 92, 98, 177
Committee for Medical Specialty Councils (CONACEM), 111
community health care units, 173
complaints procedures, 58, 68, 71t, 72, 177
complementary and alternative medicine, 156–7
Comprehensive Health Care Model (MAIS), 127, 132
computed tomography (CT) equipment, 108t
CONACEM (Committee for Medical Specialty Councils), 111
CONACYT (National Science and Technology Council), 35–6, 68, 178
CONADIC (National Commission against Addictions), 126
CONAMED (National Commission for Medical Arbitration), 58, 68, 72, 177
CONAPO (National Council on Population), 46, 49
CONAR (Council for Self-Regulation and Advertisement Ethics), 46

CONASUPO (National Company for Subsidies for the Population), 26
CONEVAL (National Council for the Evaluation of Social Development Policy), 48, 178
Confederation of Chambers of Industry of Mexico (CONCAMIN), 41–2
Confederation of National Chambers of Commerce and Tourism (CONCANACO-SERVYTUR), 41–2
conjunctivitis, 15, 16t
constitutional health rights, 17, 20, 27, 49, 52, 158, 190
consultation rooms adjacent to pharmacies (CAF), 93, 146, 147–8
convergence, 166, 168
Coordinating Commission for Negotiating the Price of Medicines and other Health Inputs (CCPNMIS), 41, 66
Coordinating Unit for Linkage and Social Participation, 34
COPLAMAR (General Coordination of the National Plan for Depressed Zones and Marginalized Groups), 26–7, 29
corporatism, 37–42, 192–3
corruption, 9, 44, 159, 165, 166, 173
cost containment, 30, 41
Council for Ethics and Transparency of the Pharmaceutical Industry (CETIFARMA), 67, 123
Council for Self-Regulation and Advertisement Ethics (CONAR), 46
COVID-19 pandemic, 195–9; about, 195; economic impacts, 195–6; hospital capacity, 197–8; monitoring and surveillance, 196–7; policy and, 198–9
cross-border health care, 73–6; migrant workers, 73; policy initiatives, 74–5; service utilization, 75–6
cuota social (social allocation), 60

day care, 140–1
death. *See* mortality
decentralization, of health system, 9, 27–8, 37, 43–5, 170
Defence. *See* Secretariat of National Defence (SEDENA)
de la Madrid, Miguel, 27

dengue, 131

dental care, 156

dentists, 113t, 116, 121, 156

diabetes: accessibility and coverage issues, 163, 179, 180–1, 188; as cause of death, 1, 11, 12, 12t, 188; economic burden of, 12, 13, 14; equity of outcomes and, 186; generic drugs and, 147; information technology and, 110; morbidity rates, 16t; national and intersectoral strategies, 46–7, 130–1; quality of care and, 188

Diagnosis Related Groups (DRGs) payment method, 91, 97t, 98

diarrhoeal diseases, 12, 12t, 186

Díaz Ordaz, Gustavo, 26

DIF (National System for Integral Family Development), 111, 128, 148

Directorate for Traditional Medicine and Intercultural Development (DMTDI), 156–7

Doctors Without Borders, 155

duodenitis, 16t

Durango, 105t, 114f, 117f, 154, 162

Echeverría Álvarez, Luis, 26

education: demographic indicators, 3t; for health workers, 119–22, 120t

efficiency, 187–9; allocative efficiency, 187–8; and health expenditures and life expectancy, 187, 187f; information technology and, 110; Seguro Popular and, 163–4; technical efficiency, 188–9

ELCOS (Labor and Social Co-responsibility Survey), 151

elderly, 128, 136, 140–1, 150

electronic health records (ECE), 109

electronic medical records (EMRs), 108, 167–8

emergency care, 141–2, 174

ENARM (National Exam for Medical Residency Candidates), 111

ENCODAT (National Survey of Drug, Alcohol and Tobacco Consumption), 128

ENCSOD (National Strategy for the Prevention and Control of Overweight, Obesity and Diabetes), 46–7, 130–1

ENOE (National Occupation and Employment Surveys), 112–13, 114, 115, 116, 118

ENSANUT (National Health and Nutrition Survey), 47, 48, 69, 102, 131, 136, 146, 186

Epidemiological Surveillance System of Oral Pathologies (SIVEPAB), 156

epidemiology: National Epidemiological Surveillance System (SINAVE), 48, 49, 126, 131–2

equity: of health care outcomes, 185–7; information technology and, 110; Seguro Popular and, 164–5

exchange agreements, high-specialty, 139, 166, 167

expenditure, health, 78–85; summary, 77, 175; growth trends, 78–9, 81t; by health function and financing scheme, 82, 85t; per capita spending, 80, 81t; private expenditure, 81t, 82; public expenditure, 81t, 82, 83f, 84f; as share of GDP, 78, 78f, 79f, 81t

family planning, 10, 46, 74, 126, 135

FASSA (Health Services Contribution Fund), 60, 86, 92, 188

FCS (Carlos Slim Foundation), 47, 110, 130

Federal Commission for Economic Competition (COFECE), 66, 147

Federal Commission for the Protection Against Sanitary Risks (COFEPRIS): about, 33; palliative care and, 152, 153; pharmaceuticals and, 66, 68, 146, 147; regulatory role, 63, 111; responsibilities of, 56, 126; social insurance coverage and, 58

Federal Reference Hospitals, 36

federal solidary contribution (ASF, *Aportación Solidaria Federal*), 60, 92

Federal Treasury (Tesofe) accounts, 44

fee-for-service (FFS), 36, 97t, 98, 127

FENACOME (National Federation of Colleges of Medicine), 110–11

fertility rate, 3t, 10, 46

financial flows, 87, 88f

financing, 77–98; summary, 77; allocative efficiency, 187–8; capital stocks and investments, 100–1; catastrophic health expenditures, 29, 35, 159, 160, 161t, 162, 163, 175, 181, 181f, 191; collection and pooling, 91; cost containment, 30, 41;

expenditure, 78–85, 175; from federal government, 34–6; financial protection, 181–2; for non-insured, 60–2; other sources of, 97; out-of-pocket payments, 92–3, 94f; payment mechanisms, 97–8, 97t; purchasing and purchaser–provider relations, 91–2; reform consensus, 169–70, 174; regulation and governance of payers, 59–63; responsibilities for, 51t; revenue sources and financing flows, 86–7, 88f; social insurance institutions, 39, 59–60, 89; statutory financing system, 88–91, 89f; System for Social Protection in Health and, 90, 160–2, 161t, 163–4, 165–6; voluntary health insurance, 94–7. *See also* out-of-pocket payments; private health insurance

food: assistance program, 46; diabetes, obesity and overweight strategies and, 46–7; insecurity, 1, 14

Fortalecimiento de la Atención Médica Program (formerly Mobile Medical Units), 102, 135

FOSISS (Sectoral Fund for Research in Health and Social Security), 35–6, 178

Fox Quezada, Vicente, 8, 29, 30

FPGC (Protection Fund for Catastrophic Health Expenditures), 35, 61, 62, 90, 98, 111, 139, 163, 171

Funsalud (Mexican Health Foundation), 144, 171

gamma cameras, 108t

gastritis, 16t

gender: life expectancy and, 9–10, 10t; mortality and, 10t, 11

General Agreement for Interinstitutional Collaboration for the Care of Obstetric Emergencies, 142

General Audit of the Federation (ASFed), 61

General Coordination of the National Plan for Depressed Zones and Marginalized Groups (COPLAMAR), 26–7, 29

General Directorate for Health Information (DGIS), 47, 49

General Directorate for Health Planning and Development (DGPLADES), 65, 101, 156

General Directorate for Health Promotion (DGPS), 125

General Directorate for Health Quality and Education (DGCES), 61, 63, 65, 139–40

General Directorate for Performance Evaluation (DGED), 48, 49, 178

General Directorate of Epidemiology, 49

General Directorate of Reproductive Health (DGSR), 126

General Health Board, 139, 164

General Health Council (GHC): about, 33, 34; FPGC coverage and, 90; non-insured and, 61; pharmaceuticals and, 65, 146; public participation and, 177; regulation of providers, 63–4; responsibilities of, 19, 52, 55–6

General Health Law: on complementary and alternative medicine, 157; on financing, 35; generic drugs and, 66; on medical specialists, 111; on National Health System, 158; non-insured and, 32, 60, 61; on organization and governance, 27–8, 30, 33, 36, 52–3, 54, 55, 56, 158; on palliative care, 151; on patient rights, 70; on person-centred care, 68; public expenditures and, 82; social insurance institutions and, 58; System for Social Protection in Health (SPSS) and, 29, 61

General Social Development Law, 178

generic drugs, 66, 146–7

geography and sociodemography, 1–4; African ancestry, people with, 2; climate and natural disasters, 4; demographic ageing, 1, 4; Indigenous peoples, 2, 26, 156–7; landmass and borders, 1–2; map, 3f; migration, internal and external, 4; population and demographic indicators, 2, 3t, 4, 10

gingivitis, 15, 16t

governance. *See* organization and governance

Guanajuato, 105t, 114f, 117f, 161

Guerrero: complementary and alternative medicine, 157; general physicians, 114f; Healthcare Access and Quality (HAQ) Index, 182; health system outcomes, 186; hospital beds, 105t; infant mortality, 11,

185; life expectancy, 10; medical specialists, 117f; mental health care, 155; social development, 10

Health, Education and Nutrition Programme (PROGRESA), 29, 46
health administrators, 118
Healthcare Access and Quality (HAQ) Index, 182, 183f
Health Care Associated Infections (HAIs), 131–2
Health Coordination Unit, 27
health information systems, 18, 47–9, 99, 108–10, 174, 179, 192
Health of Mexicans annual reports, 47–8
health promotion, 69, 74–5, 125, 128, 132, 191
Health Services Contribution Fund (FASSA), 60, 86, 92, 188
health technology, 65, 106, 108t
health workers. *See* human resources
Healthy Environments and Communities Programme, 128
heart diseases. *See* acute myocardial infarction; ischaemic heart disease
helminthiasis, 15, 16t
hepatitis A, 15, 16t
hepatitis B, 16t, 129
Hidalgo: complementary and alternative medicine, 157; general physicians, 114f; hospital beds, 105t; medical specialists, 117f; mental health care, 154; System for Social Protection in Health and, 92, 98, 165
High Specialty Hospitals, 36, 106, 122, 138, 139
high-specialty regional reference hospitals (HRAE), 100
HIV/AIDS, 12t, 15, 16t, 126, 131
homeopathy, 144t, 157
homicide (men), 12t, 13
Hospital Epidemiological Surveillance Network (RHOVE), 131–2
hospitals: accreditation, 139; capital stocks and investments, 100–1; care provision in, 138; COVID-19 pandemic and, 197–8; Federal Reference Hospitals, 36; High Specialty Hospitals, 36, 106, 122, 138, 139; high-specialty regional

reference hospitals (HRAE), 100; hospital beds, 104–6, 104t, 105t, 107t; hospital units, 102–4, 103t; Integral Hospitals, 157; organization and governance, 64; portability and convergence reforms, 166
Hospital Transition Villas, 154
Human Development Index (HDI), 10, 104, 186
human papillomavirus vaccine, 186
human resources, 110–23; summary, 99; career paths, 122–3; COVID-19 pandemic and, 198; density statistics, 112–13, 113t, 114, 116, 118, 118f; dentists, 113t, 116, 121, 156; general physicians, 43, 113t, 114–15, 114f, 115f; health administrators, 118; laboratory professionals, 121; medical malpractice, 72; medical specialists, 43, 111, 113t, 115–16, 117f, 121–2; nurses, 118, 118f, 119, 120; nutritionists, 121; organization and governance of physicians, 64; pharmacists, 121; planning and registration, 110–12; professional mobility, 119; psychiatrists, 155; psychologists, 121; public vs. private sector employment, 112; salaries, 112; System for Social Protection in Health (SPSS) and, 164–5; training, 119–22, 120t; unions and pensions, 38, 189; workforce trends, 112–18
hypertension, 12t, 16t, 110, 147, 149, 180–1

immunizations. *See* vaccinations
IMSS. *See* Mexican Social Insurance Institute (IMSS)
IMSS–Bienestar, 27, 32, 58, 92, 101, 103t, 104t
INAI (National Institute for Transparency and Access to Public Information and Data Protection), 176
INAPAM (National Institute for Older Persons), 141, 150
indemnity insurance, 18, 19–20, 59, 62, 94, 95, 96, 97
INDICAS (National System for Quality of Care Indicators), 139–40
Indigenous peoples, 2, 26, 156–7
INDRE (Institute of Epidemiological Diagnosis and Reference), 131

INEGI (National Institute of Statistics and Geography), 47, 49, 112, 144, 150
infant mortality, 2, 10t, 11, 185
influenza, 131, 186
information technology (IT), 108–10. *See also* health information systems
infrastructure. *See* physical resources
inpatient care, 50–1t, 94f
INSABI. *See* Institute for Health for Wellbeing (INSABI)
INSS (National Institute of Social Insurance), 21–3
Institute for Health for Wellbeing (INSABI): benefits package, 65; establishment and purpose, 31, 32, 53, 159, 170; financing for non-insured, 44–5, 62; funding from, 35; patient information and, 69; patient rights and, 70; states and, 36–7; transparency and accountability, 177
Institute for Social Security and Services for State Employees (ISSSTE): summary, 17; benefits and service provision, 39; capital stocks and investments, 100; collection and pooling, 91; complementary and alternative medicine, 157; coverage and participation, 37, 86, 89; COVID-19 pandemic and, 198; dental care, 156; establishment, 25; financing, 39, 59–60; governance, 37–8, 42, 45; health research, 178; health technologies, evaluation of, 65; hospital care and beds, 103t, 104t, 138, 166; informal caregivers, 151; patient information and, 69; pharmaceuticals, 146; primary care clinics, 101; private insurance and, 43; public health, 126–7; purchasing and, 91–2; rehabilitation, 149; specialized outpatient care, 136
Institute of Epidemiological Diagnosis and Reference (INDRE), 131
Institutional Revolutionary Party (PRI), 8–9, 168
insurance. *See* indemnity insurance; private health insurance; social insurance institutions
Integral Hospitals, 157

Integrated Health Programmes (PrevenIMSS), 126, 134
Integrated Mental Health Centres (UNEMES-CISAME), 155
integration, 110, 139, 191, 194
Inter-American Development Bank, 110
Interinstitutional Commission for the Training of Human Resources for Health (CIFRHS), 111–12
intermediate care, 125, 149
International Covenant on Economic, Social and Cultural Rights, 49
intersectorality, 45–7
intestinal infections, 15, 16t
ischaemic heart disease, 1, 11, 12–13, 12t
ISSSTE. *See* Institute for Social Security and Services for State Employees (ISSSTE)

Jalisco: general physicians, 114, 114f; health system development, 19; hospital beds, 105t; medical education, 120; medical specialists, 117f; mental health care, 154; population, 2; private hospitals, 104
Joint Commission International, 63

kidney diseases, 11, 12, 14, 30, 91

Labor and Social Co-responsibility Survey (ELCOS), 151
Laboratories to Support Epidemiological Surveillance (LAVE), 131
laboratory professionals, 121
labour mobility, 61, 188
Laurell, Asa Cristina, 53
Law on Insurance and Surety Institutions, 94, 96
Leave Healthy, Return Healthy Program (VSRS), 74–5
Legal Department, 34
LESP (State Public Health Laboratories), 131
licensing. *See* accreditation
life expectancy, 9–10, 10t, 185, 187, 187f
long-term care, 125, 150–1
López Mateos, Adolfo, 25
López Obrador, Andrés Manuel, 8–9, 53, 73, 97, 159, 169, 170, 176, 194, 196
López Portillo, José, 26, 27

magnetic resonance imaging (MRI) equipment, 108t

MAIS (Comprehensive Health Care Model), 127, 132

malnutrition, 14, 190

malpractice, medical, 72

mammograms and mammograph equipment, 108t, 186

Marginalization Index, 186

Master Plan for Physical Infrastructure for Health (PMI), 65, 101, 157

maternal health, 109, 126, 142

maternal mortality, 11, 166, 186

medical specialists, 43, 111, 113t, 115–16, 117f, 121–2

medical specialty councils, 63, 64, 111

Medical Specialty Units (UNEMES), 136–7

mental health, 14–15, 73, 125, 126, 153–5

Mental Health Action Programme, 155

Mexican Association of Faculties and Schools of Medicine (AMFEM), 119, 120

Mexican Association of Hospitals (AMH), 64

Mexican Association of Innovative Pharmaceutical Industry (AMIIF), 67, 68

Mexican Association of Interchangeable Generic Medicines (AMEGI), 68

Mexican Consortium of Hospitals, 64

Mexican Council for Accreditation of Medical Education (COMAEM), 119

Mexican Declaration on Psychiatric Restructuring, 154

Mexican Health Foundation (Funsalud), 144, 171

Mexican Health Promotion Directorship, 74

Mexican Observatory of Non-Communicable Diseases, 130

Mexican Petroleum Company (PEMEX): about, 37, 45; COVID-19 pandemic and, 198; financing, 86, 91; hospital accreditation, 139; hospital beds and units, 103t, 104t; primary care clinics, 101; specialized outpatient care, 138

Mexican Pharmaceutical Consortium (CFM), 67, 68

Mexican Social Insurance Institute (IMSS): summary, 17; accessibility issues, 179; benefits and service provision, 38–9, 40t; capital stocks and investments, 100; career paths, 122; collection and pooling, 91; complaints procedures, 72; cost containment, 41; coverage and participation, 37, 86, 89, 169; day care, 141; decentralization and, 28; electronic health records, 109; electronic medical records, 168; establishment and development, 18, 23–4; exchange agreements and, 167; financing, 59–60; governance, 37–8, 41–2, 45, 58, 191; health research, 178–9; health technologies, evaluation of, 65; hospital care and beds, 103t, 104t, 166; information technology and, 109; medical specialists, 122; mental health care, 155; Migrant Programme, 74; neoliberal reforms and, 29; patient choice, 69–70; patient information, 69; patient rights, 70; pharmaceuticals, 145, 146; primary care clinics, 101; private insurance and, 43, 97; public health programs, 126; purchasing and, 91–2; reform consensus, 172, 194; rehabilitation, 148–9; segmentation and, 24–5, 26–7, 191; Seguro Popular and, 166; specialized outpatient care, 136; transparency and accountability, 176; unions and pensions, 38, 189

Mexico: summary, 1; climate and natural disasters, 4; demographic ageing, 1, 4; economic context, 4–5, 6t; geography, 1–2; health status overview, 9–16; Indigenous peoples, 2, 26, 156–7; map, 3f; migration, internal and external, 4; political context, 1, 6–9; population and demographic indicators, 2, 3t, 10. *See also* Mexico, health system

Mexico (state): general physicians, 114; health spending inequalities, 161, 162; hospital beds, 105t; internal migration and, 4; medical specialists, 117f; mental health care, 154; population, 2

Mexico, health system: assessment of, 175–89; conclusions, 190–4; constitutional health rights, 17, 20, 27, 49, 52, 158, 190; corporatism, 37–42, 192–3; COVID-19 pandemic and, 195–9; financing, 77–98; historical background, 18–31; organization and governance,

17–18, 32–76; physical and human resources, 99–123; reforms, 158–74, 193–4; service provision, 124–57. *See also specific topics*

Mexico City: COVID-19 pandemic and, 195; general physicians, 114, 114f; Healthcare Access and Quality (HAQ) Index, 182; health spending inequalities, 161; hospitals and hospital beds, 100, 104, 105t, 106; infant mortality, 11, 185; life expectancy, 10; medical education, 120; medical specialists, 116, 117f; mental health care, 155; National Institutes of Health and Federal Reference Hospitals in, 36; Physician in your Home Programme, 136; population, 2

Michoacán de Ocampo, 105t, 114f, 117f, 157, 161

MIDO-Mi Salud (app), 110, 130

migrant workers, 47, 73

Miguel Hidalgo Model of Mental Health Care, 153–4

Millennium Development Goals, 166, 186

Ministry of Commerce, 66, 67

Ministry of Education, 47, 110, 111, 119

Ministry of Foreign Affairs, 75

Ministry of Health (MoH): summary, 18, 158, 159; accessibility issues, 179–80; capital planning and investments, 100–1; complaints and, 68, 72; complementary and alternative medicine, 157; cross-border health care and, 75; decentraliza-tion and, 28; dental care, 156; electronic health records, 109; electronic medical records, 168; financing and, 35–6, 59, 61; governance and organization, 33–4, 39; health information systems and, 47–9; health research, 178–9; health technol-ogies, evaluation of, 65; hospitals and beds, 63, 102, 103t, 104t, 138; human resources planning, 111; information technology and, 109; integration and, 139; intermediate care, 149; intersectoral programs, 47; mental health care, 155; overweight, obesity, and diabetes, 46–7, 130–1; pharmaceuticals, 146; primary care clinics, 101; Programme for Healthy Environments and Communities, 46;

public health, 125–6, 128; reforms and, 194; responsibilities and regulatory reach, 32, 53, 54–5, 191; Special Health Insurance Institutions (ISES) and, 63; specialized outpatient care, 136; telehealth, 109, 138; transparency and accountability, 176–7

Ministry of Health and Assistance (SSA), 24, 27

Ministry of the Public Function, 72

Ministry of the Treasury and Public Credit, 42, 46, 58, 66, 67, 111

Ministry of Welfare, 46

morbidity, 13–15, 15t, 16t

Morelos, 105t, 114f, 117f, 162

Morena (Movement for National Regeneration party), 8–9

mortality: causes of, 1, 11–13, 12t, 184; infant mortality, 2, 10t, 11, 185; maternal mortality, 11, 166, 186; palliative care, 125, 151–3, 152t; rates of, 10t, 11; work-related accidents, 15t

motor vehicle (traffic) accidents, 11, 12t, 13, 15t, 47

Movement for National Regeneration party (Morena), 8–9

Multidimensional Measurement of Poverty, 186

municipal governments, 7, 128

National Academy of Medicine (ANM), 19, 111, 122

National Action Party (PAN), 8–9, 168

National Agreement Towards the Universalization of Health Services (*Acuerdo Nacional hacia la Universalización de los Servicios de Salud*), 139

National Association of Drug Distributors (ANADIM), 145t

National Association of Pharmaceutical Manufacturers (ANAFAM), 68, 144

National Association of Pharmacies of Mexico (ANAFARMEX), 145t

National Association of Private Hospitals (ANHP), 64

National Association of Regional Pharmaceutical Companies (ANEFAR), 145t

National Basic Health Information System (SINBA), 48–9, 109, 110, 192

National Centre for Pharmacovigilance, 143

National Centre for the Health of Children and Adolescents (CENSIA), 126

National Centre for the Prevention and Control of HIV/AIDS (CENSIDA), 126

National Centre of Technological Excellence in Health (CENETEC), 65

National Chamber of the Pharmaceutical Industry (Canifarma), 67–8

National College of Physicians (CMM), 64, 110–11

National Commission against Addictions (CONADIC), 126

National Commission for Human Rights (CNDH), 68

National Commission for Medical Arbitration (CONAMED), 58, 68, 72, 177

National Commission for National Institutes of Health and High Specialty Hospitals (CINSHAE), 34, 36, 111, 138

National Company for Subsidies for the Population (CONASUPO), 26

National Council for the Evaluation of Social Development Policy (CONEVAL), 48, 178

National Council on Population (CONAPO), 46, 49

National Defence. *See* Secretariat of National Defence (SEDENA)

National Epidemiological Surveillance System (SINAVE), 48, 49, 126, 131–2

National Exam for Medical Residency Candidates (ENARM), 111

National Federation of Colleges of Medicine (FENACOME), 110–11

National Health Accounts Information System (SICUENTAS), 48

National Health and Nutrition Survey (ENSANUT), 47, 48, 69, 102, 131, 136, 146, 186

National Health Council, 28, 34, 45, 177

National Health Information System (SINAIS), 48

National Health System (NHS), 28, 33, 55, 158, 190. *See also* Mexico, health system

National Health Weeks, 132

National Institute for Older Persons (INAPAM), 141, 150

National Institute for Transparency and Access to Public Information and Data Protection (INAI), 176

National Institute of Rehabilitation, 148

National Institute of Social Insurance (INSS), 21–3

National Institute of Statistics and Geography (INEGI), 47, 49, 112, 144, 150

National Institutes of Health, 27, 36, 138, 139, 178

National Law of Access to Public Information, 176

National Medical Centres, 138

National Mid-Way Health and Nutrition Survey, 129

National Network of Public Health Laboratories (RNLSP), 131

National Occupation and Employment Surveys (ENOE), 112–13, 114, 115, 116, 118

National Programme of Solidarity through Community Cooperation, 26

National Researchers System, 178

National Science and Technology Council (CONACYT), 35–6, 68, 178

National Strategy for the Prevention and Control of Overweight, Obesity and Diabetes (ENCSOD), 46–7, 130–1

National Survey of Addictions, 128

National Survey of Drug, Alcohol and Tobacco Consumption (ENCODAT), 128

National System for Certification of Medical Care Establishments (SiNaCEAM), 63–4, 139

National System for Integral Family Development (DIF), 111, 128, 148

National System for Quality of Care Indicators (INDICAS), 139–40

National System of Health Records, 156

National System of Medical Residencies, 111–12

National Union of Pharmacy Entrepreneurs (UNEFARM), 145t

Navy. *See* Secretariat of the Navy (SEMAR)

Nayarit, 105t, 114f, 117f

neonatal screening, 128, 129–30. *See also* prenatal care

nephropathy, 14. *See also* kidney diseases

New Generation Medical Insurance programme, 87

non-insured: summary, 175, 191; funding for, 60–2, 188; health services for, 44–5, 182; hospital units and beds, 103t, 104t; private health care and, 42. *See also* Institute for Health for Wellbeing (INSABI); System for Social Protection in Health (SPSS) and Seguro Popular

Nuevo León: general physicians, 114, 114f; Healthcare Access and Quality (HAQ) Index, 182; health spending inequalities, 162; hospital beds, 105t; IMSS and, 25; internal migration and, 4; medical specialists, 116, 117f; private hospitals, 104

nurses, 118, 118f, 119, 120

nutritionists, 121

Oaxaca: complementary and alternative medicine, 157; general physicians, 114f; Healthcare Access and Quality (HAQ) Index, 182; health spending inequalities, 162; health system outcomes, 186; hospital beds, 105t; medical specialists, 117f; mental health care, 154; municipalities in, 6; telehealth, 109

obesity. *See* overweight and obesity

Obregón, Álvaro, 19, 20, 21

obstetric emergencies, 139, 142

occupational accidents and diseases, 15t

opioid medications, 153

Oportunidades (now Bienestar), 46

organization and governance, 17–76; summary, 17–18, 32, 33f; accountability and transparency, 176–7; background, 18–31; conditional cash transfers, 29; constitutional health rights, 17, 20, 27, 49, 52, 158, 190; corporatism, 37–42, 192–3; decentralization and centralization, 9, 27–8, 37, 43–5, 166, 170; federal level, 33–6; health information systems, 47–9, 108–10, 174, 179, 192; intersectorality, 45–7; performance monitoring and research, 178–9; person-centred care,

68–76; principal policy orientations, 49, 52–3; private sector, 42–3; public health, 125–8; public participation, 177; reform consensus, 170–2; regulation and planning, 49–68; responsibility for specific health system functions, 49, 50–1t; segmentation, 24–5, 26–7, 159, 168–9, 170–1, 175–6, 190–1; state level, 36–7; transparency and accountability, 176–7

Organs for Internal Control (OIC), 34, 72

Ortiz Rubio, Pascual, 21

outcomes, health care, 185–7

out-of-pocket payments: about, 92–3, 94f; pharmaceuticals and, 69; private sector and, 43; rates of, 163, 175, 181, 190–1; reform consensus, 170; Seguro Popular and, 93, 165; as share of health expenditure, 30, 81t, 82, 86, 87

outpatient care: accessibility issues, 179; expenditure by health function and financing scheme, 82, 85t; mental health care, 155; out-of-pocket expenses and, 94f; payment mechanisms, 97t; private sector and, 102, 136; specialized outpatient care, 136–8

overweight and obesity, 1, 13, 15t, 16t, 46–7, 121, 130–1

PABI (Self-Regulation of Food and Non-Alcoholic Drink Advertisement Directed to Child Audiences), 46

palliative care, 125, 151–3, 152t

PAN (National Action Party), 8–9, 168

Pan American Health Organization (PAHO), 66, 74, 196

patient-centred care. *See* person-centred care

patient choice, 18, 69–70, 135, 167

patient information, 69

patient pathways, 132–4

patient registration, 167

patient rights, 70, 71t

Patient's Charter, 68–9

payment mechanisms, 77, 97–8, 97t, 163

PEMEX. *See* Mexican Petroleum Company (PEMEX)

Peña Nieto, Enriquo, 53, 168–9, 176

pensions, 38, 60, 169, 172, 189

performance monitoring, 178

periodontal disease, 16t

person-centred care, 68–76; complaints procedures, 58, 68, 71t, 72, 177; constitutional and legal basis, 68–9; cross-border health care, 73–6; patient choice, 18, 69–70, 135, 167; patient information, 69; patient rights, 70, 71t; public participation, 177

pharmaceuticals, 143–8; summary, 124–5; approval process, 65, 146; cost containment, 41; dispensing, 146; distribution, 145, 145t; generic drugs, 66, 146–7; integration of prescription and dispensing, 147–8; market, 144–5, 144t; opioid medications, 153; patient choice and, 69–70; policy development, 143; quality of care, 184–5; reform consensus, 174; regulation, government, 66–7; regulation, self-, 67–8; responsibility for, 50–1t; System for Social Protection in Health (SPSS) and, 165; training, 121

pharmacists, 121

physical activity, 13–14

physical resources, 100–10; summary, 99; capital stock and investments, 100–1; health information systems and information technology, 18, 47–9, 99, 108–10, 174, 179, 192; hospital beds, 104–6, 104t, 105t, 107t; hospital units, 102–4, 103t; primary care, 101–2; technical efficiency, 189; technological equipment, 65, 106, 108t

Physician in your Home Programme, 136

physicians: general physicians, 43, 113t, 114–15, 114f, 115f; medical specialists, 43, 111, 113t, 115–16, 117f, 121–2; organization and governance, 64

planning. See regulation and planning

PMI (Master Plan for Physical Infrastructure for Health), 65, 101, 157

pneumonia, 15, 16t

Policy for Free Health Services and Medicines, 31, 62, 159

population and population growth, 2, 3t, 10

population policy, 46

portability, 166–8

Portes Gil, Emilio, 21

positron emission tomography (PET) equipment, 108t

poverty: about, 1, 2, 5, 6t; action against via IMSS, 26–7, 29; COVID-19 pandemic and, 196; health care access and, 182; intersectoral programs for, 46; monitoring, 178; System for Social Protection in Health (SPSS) and, 160

pregnancy, teen, 46, 184

prenatal care, 135, 136, 184, 186. See also neonatal screening

PrevenIMSS (Integrated Health Programmes), 126, 134

Preventive Care Model (PrevenISSSTE), 126–7

PRI (Institutional Revolutionary Party), 8–9, 168

primary care: about, 124, 135–6, 137t; accreditation and evaluation, 139–40, 140f; electronic health and medical records, 109, 168; infrastructure, 101–2

private health insurance, 94–7; summary, 32, 77; governance and public policy, 62–3, 96–7; market behaviour, 96; market structure, 95; payment mechanisms and, 98; role and size, 94–5; as share of health expenditure, 81t, 82, 87; social insurance institutions and, 43; types of, 59

private sector: about, 32, 42–3; accessibility issues and, 180; capital stocks and investments, 99, 100–1; COVID-19 pandemic and, 198; dental care, 156; hospitals, 102, 103t, 138; human resources and career paths, 111, 122–3; information technology, 109–10; primary care, 102–4; reform consensus, 171–2; rehabilitation, 149

professional mobility, 119

Programme for Healthy Environments and Communities, 46

PROGRESA (Health, Education and Nutrition Programme), 29, 46

Prospera (now Bienestar), 46

prostate: cancer, 12t; hyperplasia of, 16t

Protection Fund for Catastrophic Health Expenditures (FPGC), 35, 61, 62, 90, 98, 111, 139, 163, 171

providers and provision: at federal level, 36; payment mechanisms and, 77, 97–8, 97t, 163; purchasing and purchaser–provider

relations, 91–2; regulation and governance, 63–4

psychiatrists, 155

psychologists, 121

public health, 125–32; development of,
20; governance and organization, 50–1t,
125–8; National Epidemiological
Surveillance System (SINAVE), 48,
49, 126, 131–2; neonatal screening,
128, 129–30; overweight, obesity, and
diabetes, 46–7, 130–1; reform consensus,
173; sectoral coordination, 132; tobacco
regulation, 128; vaccinations, 126, 128,
129, 132, 135, 186

public participation, 177

public–private services agreements (PPS), 100

Puebla: complementary and alternative
medicine, 157; general physicians, 114f;
health spending inequalities, 161, 162;
health system outcomes, 186; hospital
beds, 105t; medical specialists, 117f

quality, health care, 51t, 75, 110, 139–40,
140f, 174, 184–5

Querétaro, 4, 105t, 114f, 117f, 157

Quintana Roo, 105t, 114f, 117f, 186

Radar CI-Salud (app), 109

radiation therapy equipment, 108t

Red Cross, 141, 142

reforms, 158–74; summary, 158–9; consensus on future developments, 169–74,
193–4; exchange agreements, 139, 166,
167; portability and convergence, 166–8;
segmentation persistence despite, 168–9,
170–1. *See also* Institute for Health for
Wellbeing (INSABI); System for Social
Protection in Health (SPSS) and Seguro
Popular

regulation and planning, 49–68; accreditation, 50t, 61, 63–4, 119, 122, 139, 171–2;
federal level, 54–6; human resources,
110–12; for non-insured, 60–2; of payers,
59–63; of pharmaceuticals, 66–8; principal policy orientations, 49, 52–3; private
health insurance, 62–3, 96; private sector
and, 171–2; of providers, 63–4; responsibility for, 50–1t; of services and goods,

64–5; social insurance institutions, 58,
59–60; state level, 56–8; tobacco, 128

rehabilitation, 125, 148–9

Repatriation Programme for Seriously Ill
Nationals, 75

reproductive health, 126, 184, 198

REPSS. *See* State Regimens for Social
Protection in Health (REPSS)

research, health, 35–6, 138, 174, 178–9

respiratory infections, 12, 12t, 15, 16t

revenue, sources of, 86–7

RHOVE (Hospital Epidemiological
Surveillance Network), 131–2

RNLSP (National Network of Public
Health Laboratories), 131

Ruiz Cortínez, Adolfo, 25

SAEH (Automated Hospital Discharge
Subsystem), 48

Salinas de Gortari, Carlos, 8, 29

Salud Pública de México (journal), 178–9

Sanitary Jurisdictions, 127

San Luis Potosí, 105t, 106, 114f, 117f

School Health Programme, 156

Secretariat of National Defence
(SEDENA): about, 37; financing, 86,
91; hospital beds and units, 103t, 104t;
primary care clinics, 101; rehabilitation,
149; telehealth, 138

Secretariat of the Navy (SEMAR): about,
37; complementary and alternative
medicine, 157; financing, 86, 91; hospital
beds and units, 103t, 104t; primary care
clinics, 101

Sectoral Fund for Basic Research, 178

Sectoral Fund for Research in Health and
Social Security (FOSISS), 35–6, 178

Sectoral Health Plan 2019–2024, 173

SEDENA. *See* Secretariat of National
Defence (SEDENA)

segmentation, 24–5, 26–7, 159, 168–9,
170–1, 175–6, 190–1

Seguro Popular. *See* System for Social
Protection in Health (SPSS) and Seguro
Popular

Self-Regulation of Food and Non-
Alcoholic Drink Advertisement Directed
to Child Audiences (PABI), 46

sentinel model, 196
service provision, 124–57; summary,
    124–5; by caregivers, 151; comple-
    mentary and alternative medicine,
    156–7; day care, 140–1; dental care,
    156; emergency care, 141–2; hospital
    care, 138; integration of, 139; inter-
    mediate care, 149; long-term care,
    150–1; mental health, 153–5; National
    Epidemiological Surveillance System
    (SINAVE), 48, 49, 126, 131–2; neonatal
    screening, 128, 129–30; overweight,
    obesity, and diabetes, 46–7, 130–1;
    palliative care, 151–3, 152t; patient
    pathways, 132–4; pharmaceuticals,
    143–8; primary and ambulatory care,
    135–6, 137t; public health, 125–32;
    quality evaluation of acute medical care,
    139–40, 140f; regulation and planning,
    64–5; rehabilitation, 148–9; specialized
    outpatient care, 136–8; tobacco regula-
    tion, 128; vaccinations, 29, 73, 126, 128,
    129, 132, 135, 186
sexual abuse, of children, 46
sexual health. *See* reproductive health
SICUENTAS (National Health Accounts
    Information System), 48
SiNaCEAM (National System for
    Certification of Medical Care
    Establishments), 63–4, 139
SINAIS (National Health Information
    System), 48
Sinaloa, 105t, 114f, 117f, 182
SINAVE (National Epidemiological
    Surveillance System), 48, 49, 126, 131–2
SINBA (National Basic Health
    Information System), 48–9, 109, 110, 192
SINERHIAS (System for Health Care
    Equipment, Human Resources and
    Infrastructure), 48
SIVEPAB (Epidemiological Surveillance
    System of Oral Pathologies), 156
smoking, 14, 15t. *See also* tobacco regulation
social allocation (*cuota social*), 60
social determinants of health, 14, 46, 173
social insurance institutions: summary, 17,
    18, 88; accessibility issues, 179; collection

and pooling, 91; contractual relations
    with states and providers, 51t; cost
    containment, 41; coverage and benefits
    package, 38–9, 64–5, 89; development
    of, 21–3; financial protection and, 182;
    financing, 39, 59–60, 77; governance and
    organization, 32, 41–2, 45, 191; health
    research and, 35–6; patient informa-
    tion and, 69; patient pathways and,
    133; patient rights and, 70; payment
    mechanisms and, 98; pharmaceuticals,
    146; private insurance and, 42, 43;
    public health and, 127; purchasing and
    purchaser–provider relations, 91–2;
    regulation and, 58; rehabilitation, 148–9.
    See also Institute for Social Security
    and Services for State Employees
    (ISSSTE); Mexican Petroleum Company
    (PEMEX); Mexican Social Insurance
    Institute (IMSS); Secretariat of National
    Defence (SEDENA); Secretariat of the
    Navy (SEMAR)
Social Insurance Law, 23–4, 26, 37, 45, 52,
    58, 89, 176
sociodemography. *See* geography and
    sociodemography
socioeconomic status, 43, 93, 94f, 95, 133,
    185, 190
Sonora, 105t, 114f, 117f
Special Health Insurance Institutions
    (ISES), 62–3, 96, 97
specialists, medical, 43, 111, 113t, 115–16,
    117f, 121–2
Specialized Health Insurance, 59
Specialized Medical Units in Chronic
    Diseases (UNEMES-EC), 149
Specialized Technical Committee for
    Sectoral Health Information, 47
Specialty Clinics, 136
SPSS. *See* System for Social Protection in
    Health (SPSS) and Seguro Popular
state government solidary contribution
    (ASE), 60
State Health Councils, 28, 45
State Public Health Laboratories (LESP), 131
State Regimens for Social Protection in
    Health (REPSS): about, 37, 44, 58;

accountability and transparency, 177; financing and, 35, 59, 61–2, 98, 163; public participation, 177
Statistical and Geographic Information System, 49
suicide, 12t, 13
SUIVE (Unique Epidemiological Surveillance Information System), 48, 131
syphilis, 131
System for Health Care Equipment, Human Resources and Infrastructure (SINERHIAS), 48
System for Social Protection in Health (SPSS) and Seguro Popular: summary, 18, 77, 175, 191; capital stocks and investments, 100; coverage and benefits package, 65, 90; demand-side funding by, 165–6; development and demise, 29–31, 53, 158, 159–60; electronic health records, 109; equity and efficiency impacts, 163–5; financial impact of, 160–2, 161t; financial protection and, 181–2; financing and, 35, 36, 44, 60–1, 87, 91, 160, 171; meaning of Seguro Popular name, 52n; mental health care, 154; migrant workers and, 74; out-of-pocket expenses and, 93, 165; patient information and, 69; patient rights and, 70; payment mechanisms and, 98; Peña Nieto administration and, 169; purchasing and, 92; transparency and accountability, 176–7

Tabasco, 105t, 114f, 117f, 155, 186
Tamaulipas, 105t, 114f, 117f, 120, 154, 155, 182
technical efficiency, 188–9
technological equipment, 65, 106, 108t
telehealth and telemedicine, 108–9, 110, 138
Telethon Foundation: Teletón Children's System (SIT), 149
Tesofe (Federal Treasury) accounts, 44
Tlaxcala, 105t, 114f, 117f, 186
tobacco regulation, 128. *See also* smoking
traditional medicine, 156–7
traffic (motor vehicle) accidents, 11, 12t, 13, 15t, 47

training, for health workers, 119–22, 120t
transparency and accountability, 176–7
tuberculosis, 12t, 15, 16t, 131
21st Century Medical Insurance programme, 87

ulcers, 15, 16t
Undersecretary for Administration and Financing, 34
Undersecretary of Prevention and Health Promotion, 125
UNEFARM (National Union of Pharmacy Entrepreneurs), 145t
UNEMES (Medical Specialty Units), 136–7
UNEMES-CISAME (Integrated Mental Health Centres), 155
UNEMES-EC (Specialized Medical Units in Chronic Diseases), 149
unions, trade, 38, 189
Unique Epidemiological Surveillance Information System (SUIVE), 48, 131
Unique Health Establishment Code (CLUES), 48
United Kingdom, 23
United States of America, 20, 23, 73–5
Unit for Economic Analysis, 34
Universal Health Services Catalogue (CAUSES), 35, 61, 62, 90, 139, 146, 154, 163
universal right to health, 193–4
urinary tract infections, 15, 16t
US–Mexico Border Health Association (USMBHA), 74
US–Mexico Border Health Commission, 74

vaccinations, 29, 73, 126, 128, 129, 132, 135, 186
Veracruz de Ignacio de la Llave: complementary and alternative medicine, 157; general physicians, 114f; health spending inequalities, 162; health system outcomes, 186; hospital beds, 105t; medical specialists, 117f; mental health care, 155
voluntary health insurance. *See* private health insurance

VSRS (Leave Healthy, Return Healthy Program), 74–5

vulvovaginitis, 16t

women's health, 184. *See also* maternal health; prenatal care; reproductive health

World Bank, 29

World Health Organization (WHO), 29, 53, 152, 174

Yucatán, 19, 105t, 114f, 117f, 186

Zacatecas, 105t, 114f, 117f

Zedillo Ponce de León, Ernesto, 28, 29

The Health Systems in Transition Series

**A series of the European Observatory
on Health Systems and Policies**

The Health Systems in Transition (HiT) country reports provide an analytical description of each health system and of reform initiatives in progress or under development. They aim to provide relevant comparative information to support policy-makers and analysts in the development of health systems and reforms in the countries of the WHO European Region and beyond.

The HiTs are building blocks that can be used:

- to learn in detail about different approaches to the financing, organization and delivery of health services;
- to describe accurately the process, content and implementation of health reform programmes;
- to highlight common challenges and areas that require more in-depth analysis; and
- to provide a tool for the dissemination of information on health systems and the exchange of experiences of reform strategies between policy-makers and analysts in countries of the WHO European Region.

How to obtain a HiT

All HiTs are available as PDF files at www.healthobservatory.eu, where you can also join our listserve for monthly updates of the activities of the European Observatory on Health Systems and Policies, including new HiTs, books in our co-published series with Cambridge University Press, Policy briefs, Policy Summaries, and the Eurohealth journal.

If you would like to order a paper copy of a HiT, please contact us at: contact@obs.who.int

The publications of the
European Observatory on
Health Systems and Policies
are available at

www.healthobservatory.eu

HiT Country Reviews Published to Date

Albania
(1999, 2002^{ag})

Andorra
(2004)

Armenia
(2001^g, 2006, 2013)

Australia
(2002, 2006)

Austria
(2001^e, 2006^e, 2013^e, 2018)

Azerbaijan
(2004^g, 2010^g)

Belarus
(2008^g, 2013)

Belgium
(2000, 2007, 2010)

Bosnia and Herzegovina
(2002^g)

Bulgaria
(1999, 2003^b, 2007^g, 2012, 2018)

Canada
(2005, 2013^c)

Croatia
(1999, 2006, 2014)

Cyprus
(2004, 2012)

Czech Republic
(2000, 2005^g, 2009, 2015)

Denmark
(2001, 2007^g, 2012)

Estonia
(2000, 2004^{gi}, 2008, 2013, 2018)

Finland
(2002, 2008, 2019)

France
(2004^{cg}, 2010, 2015)

Georgia
(2002^{dg}, 2009, 2017)

Germany
(2000^e, 2004^{eg}, 2014^e)

Greece
(2010, 2017)

Hungary
(1999, 2004, 2011)

Iceland
(2003, 2014)

Ireland
(2009)

Israel
(2003, 2009, 2015)

Italy
(2001, 2009, 2014)

Japan
(2009)

Kazakhstan
(1999^g, 2007^g, 2012)

Kyrgyzstan
(2000^g, 2005^g, 2011^g)

Latvia
(2001, 2008, 2012, 2019)

Lithuania
(2000, 2013)

Luxembourg
(1999, 2015)

Malta
(1999, 2014, 2017)

Mongolia
(2007)

Netherlands
(2004^g, 2010, 2016)

New Zealand
(2001*)

Norway
(2000, 2006, 2013, 2020)

Poland
(1999, 2005^k, 2011, 2019)

Portugal
(1999, 2004, 2007, 2011, 2017)

Republic of Korea
(2009*)

Republic of Moldova
(2002^g, 2008^g, 2012)

Romania
(2000^f, 2008, 2016)

Russian Federation
(2003^g, 2011^g)

Serbia
(2019)

Slovakia
(2000, 2004, 2011, 2016)

Slovenia
(2002, 2009, 2016)

Spain
(2000h, 2006, 2010, 2018)

Sweden
(2001, 2005, 2012)

Switzerland
(2000, 2015)

Tajikistan
(2000, 2010^g, 2016)

The former Yugoslav Republic of Macedonia
(2000, 2006, 2017)

Turkey
(2002^{gi}, 2011^i)

Turkmenistan
(2000)

Ukraine
(2004^g, 2010^g, 2015)

United Kingdom of Great Britain and Northern Ireland
(1999^g, 2015)

United Kingdom (England)
(2011)

United Kingdom (Northern Ireland)
(2012)

United Kingdom (Scotland)
(2012)

United Kingdom (Wales)
(2012)

United States of America
(2013)

Uzbekistan
(2001^g, 2007^g, 2014^g)

Veneto Region, Italy
(2012)

All HiTs are available in English.
When noted, they are also available in other languages:

a	Albanian
b	Bulgarian
i	Estonian
c	French
d	Georgian
e	German
k	Polish
f	Romanian
g	Russian
h	Spanish
i	Turkish